Betrayed BY SELF

One Doctor's Account Of Hope, Intrigue, And Inspiration In The Face Of Psychosis

PATRICK J. MCLAUGHLIN D.O.

Contact information

For more information regarding Dr. Patrick McLaughlin, his future publications, and current practice locations, please visit: www.DoctorMcLaughlin.com. Also look for him on Facebook and Instagram.

For secure email correspondence please feel free to contact Dr. McLaughlin at DoctorMcLaughlin@protonmail.com

ISBN: 978-1-7361940-0-3

Patrick J. McLaughlin Inc.
Pismo Beach, CA

Cover design by Tami Boyce (www.tamiboyce.com)

To my parents:

Through your tireless example you have instilled in me the work ethic required to become successful and without your love and support none of this would be possible. I do apologize for all the grey hairs but according to the latest in research on genetics and behavior I can only be held responsible for 40% of those wild times.

To my son:

You are the true inspiration behind it all.
Never give up. Never doubt yourself.
Never forget how much I love you!

TABLE OF CONTENTS

BACKGROUND

The question I get asked the most is, "When did you decide to become a doctor?" So, here is the answer. Note that this reply is one that I am apprehensive to reveal, and this introduction has been removed or altered many times throughout the process of writing this book.

The hesitation I experience is regarding the underlying consideration: *Do people truly want to know about their doctors?* Is there some comfort in believing that the person responsible for your care has been nothing but golden his or her entire life? Do you really want to know that your doctor may endure the same issues that you suffer from? Doctors are bred to be professional and to perform by the book. They are instilled throughout medical school, and residency, with the belief that they are somehow above the human aspect and should act accordingly. The old adage, *you enter medical school as a person and leave as a doctor,* in itself is not far from the truth, at least in the minds of many of my colleagues, yet honestly, how aligned with reality is this notion? On the exterior, doctors may appear to be free from mental and emotional uncertainties—the epitome of health with unflawed social aspects and home lives. Fortunately, this is not true, as the hardships many of us encounter both as physicians, and in our lives lived before, enhance our capacity to relate and empathize with our patients. In similarities of struggle, which need not be exact in overall emotional content, is where we as humans align our paths of understanding to one another. When we embrace the human under the white coat, we find the line between doctor and patient to be often blurred. Within this obscured distinction is where we may find comfort in our similarities rather than trepidation from the mirror before us. The medical doctor is no different from the patient, as both are born to endure life by biological means, yet each only truly growing in purpose, and in self, by way of persistence and endurance through the adversities that life is so keen on throwing at us.

So, when did I decide to become a doctor? Here is the answer, and with it, your last chance to close this book, walk away, and remain protected from the knowledge that some doctors come not from entitled homes and families. Some come not from a lineage of physicians before them, but instead, arise from poverty, doubt, and overwhelming odds. Of course, you will get the severely abridged version of my story, simply an undefined outline, which will most likely trigger more questions than answers. In place of detailed accounts of my own historical hurdles, I chose to keep the focus of this book on the lives of the patients. However, to justly understand the personal interactions I have with patients, I find it befitting to provide some insight into the man behind the voice. This is a small but authentic offering of understanding into the struggles I personally overcame. The road was certainly not easy yet, with endurance through adversity, I was afforded the blessing of being in a position to help others.

We begin our story with a simple man devoid of hope, a man who had once attained brief success in life, employment, love, and friendship. A man who was blindsided by a moment that changed everything. It was a fraction in time, unforeseen, when all became barren. When the adrenaline regressed, he awoke to a new reality—a new awareness embodied in loss and one defined by the act of holding his uncle's lifeless body in his arms. His attempts to revive him, futile. An abrupt introduction to a world in which life could be taken much too soon.

What followed was more turmoil, and when he looked upon the wreckage, he found only emptiness within a thick cloud of ash. All direction to normality was now covered in dark grey soot, and with it, each path home evaded his perspective view. This catalyst would touch so many aspects of his life, becoming the initial crack in his dam of stability. The fracture, slowly widening, would eventually succumb to the forces—forces yearning and scratching, in desperation, to burst through. The surge that followed would be overwhelming, with the rushing waters sweeping him from his foundation of identity, attempting to drown all in a sea of distraction.

Throughout the following years, he wandered lost, entranced by nightfall and debauchery, comforted only by the music of loud pipes and nightclubs. Floating in the Las

Vegas scene, he never realized the sand of his life slowly being carried away. Opportunities inspired pitfalls, and all promises of success seemed to end in failure as the enticement of fast money and an even faster life was its own betrayal. Time continued to tick away with no resolution of fulfillment and no branches to save him from the rushing tides. Every surge of water washed away more of his sense of self and all he held dear. As the seasons passed, his losses compiled until he was destitute, deep within the rabbit hole that was now his home.

Then came the defining act of his play, and within it, a simple decision representing the most complicated of consequences. The evening was more calm than free when he found himself balanced upon a point of decisiveness engrained in reflection of future opportunities, or lack thereof. He had driven to a summit allowing him to gaze upon the house he once owned, yet still able to view the never-ending lights of the Las Vegas strip. As he stood alone, abounding with regrets of lost potential, he had all but accepted that he had been weighed and measured. The years had not been kind and he continued to suffer loss. Now devoid of all comforts, he was forced to find a reason to withstand. He thought not about the hunger from his third day without food and not of the feeling of failure that comes from being without a roof to call his own. He felt he deserved no better than he had been granted and had no reserve of faith left to draw from. He felt as there was no reason to continue to endure.

He stood solitary, focused solely on regret. A regret concerning what he could have done with his life if only he could return to his younger and more innocent self. A regret born through weakness of self and loss of drive towards a singular vision. A man beaten, yet still in possession of sufficient insight to know the significance of human determination and what is possible once that individual refuses to be the victim of their situation. An obvious notion that is much easier reflected within than acted upon.

With this regret came remorse for the wasted opportunities and overabundance of fruitless second chances. It was at this juncture, the moment that the mind steps onto the tracks of an oncoming train, that some are able to garner a swift sliver of insight. In just a fragment of a second, he asked the question, *what if*? With this question lingering unanswered, he dreamed how he would have pushed himself to become something different, someone significant, something unattainable for a boy from a low-income family. *I would have become a doctor*; he thinks to himself. It had been a lifelong daydream, and in his eyes, this was all it could ever be. It was something he had never actually said out loud as he believed such aspirations to be reserved for those in a class elite and greatly shadowing his own. He laughed in disgust for his arrogance of such a thought, as if a judge had interrupted the absurdity of his closing argument to yell out, "Guilty!"

His thoughts again slipped and began to bargain with the dullness of his own mortality. His deliberations became his voice, and he began to speak out loud. "I'm twenty-eight. I am too damn old to go chasing dreams. That's just crazy." It's unclear why his voice was now active in outright dictation of his thoughts. Maybe it is human nature to seek out another's voice during times of severe stress, and in this solitude, the only voice he could call upon was his own.

With the brain craving life and his mind bent on destruction, he again bargained. "Become a doctor? That's impossible, it's crazy, I'm nothing. I'm a loser." The pain of self-deprecation is even more agonizing when one realizes the speed at which such a phrase leaves the lips. It became obvious that this was not some foreign thought but one he had held often and an ideation of self he believed to be the truth; nonetheless, the mind remained surprised at the realization of such self-reported insignificance. At the time, he did not realize it, but "impossibility" was the representation of difficulty he needed. He assessed this random notion of implausibility and the 4,380 days of study and focus it would require. It would have to be something so challenging that he would have no time for self-doubt, nor the destructive ways enticed by distraction. It was an unintended option of chance and so provided when one finds nowhere farther to fall. This notion presented a challenge of courage, not from a point of desperation or even imposed will, but instead simply from an exclusion and reduction of rational thought.

What arose in thought next was something that seemed incongruent to the theme at hand. A coffee mug? Yes, a coffee mug. He suddenly and unexpectedly remembered this mundane object in a store from the not-too-distant past. The coffee cup was not obviously profound to him at the time, yet now, for some reason, its message was ever consuming. The morning's message of inspiration, hidden away upon this most unassuming of vessels. Its inscription read, *What Would You Attempt If You Knew You Could Not Fail?* Here, now, and without reference, he oddly finds the phrase empowering.

That phrase would replay in his mind over and over with no answer attached. With his life in a tailspin, approaching the ground with a quickness, these 11 words truly made him question his ultimate purpose. It was a vivid representation of everything involved in the current clamoring of thought. It was a mantra burdening the soul with self-reflections, yet at the same time taunting him to do something about it. He could have never comprehended the impact that simple coffee mug would have on him or its message's ultimate gravity until this moment.

In that moment and upon that mount, he would succumb to the test of a final trial and with it create a new recipe for success. One scoop of checkered past, two cups of poor decisions, a sprinkle of self-sabotage, a dash of homelessness, and finally decorate the whole damn thing in tattoos. Call it what you will—an epiphany, a sense of self-preservation, or just a continuation of crazy—but it was at that moment the decision, or better yet the challenge, to become a physician, more specifically a psychiatrist, was born. For the first time he spoke out loud of his intentions, giving them merit in accountability and as tears of rebirth began to swell, he smiled. He actually smiled, which was something he had not experienced in as long as he could remember. He smiled at a purpose more crucial than those of transitory struggles. He had found himself and acquired a realized sense of motivation that had been incarcerated beneath the soil of his feet.

That day, with only a backpack of clothes and $400, which was received from pawning his last few possessions, he lifted his leg back over his Harley and began a 12-year journey to becoming a doctor. Never looking back and never again doubting himself, he continued to work at odd jobs during nightfall, often as a bouncer or bartender, yet this time was trailed by scholarly activities of undergrad by day. He slept little, took no vacations, and studied incessantly. Yet, every single day, no matter how difficult things became, always allowing himself a few brief moments to stop—to simply stop whatever he was doing to enjoy something beautiful, something simple, and to remind himself how lucky he was to have not just life, but a life with purpose.

So, when did I decide to become a doctor? As you can see, the answer was simpler in clarification than the question posed. The decision was demanding yet uncomplicated. I knew the deficits of my attention would require a definition of success to be represented by something I truly felt was unattainable, yet I held the determination, better yet the stubbornness, to try anyway. My history of hardships, even those you will never hear me speak of, are no more unique or tortuous than those many of us have faced in life. The only details of this story that are unique lie in the fact that it was mine to overcome. In conventional description, "*I had hit rock bottom*," yet I decided to use that not as a crypt to lie in but as a solid foundation from which to rise from. I did this not alone, but with purpose. I learned in that moment of clarity that a purpose-driven life can become a rope to success, and from that point forward I thought not of myself as less-than, but instead as a future-physician.

Now I challenge you to do the same. Define your version of success, determine its path and duration, and then take the step towards a purpose-driven life. Using a woven tether of determination and clear definition of success, conquer your fears of failure and look beyond the complacency of accepting what you have been awarded. Ask yourself, "What would you attempt to do if you knew you could not fail?" When you find your answer, see yourself no longer in your current state, but that as the man or woman you will soon become. Remember, with purpose comes drive and with drive come self-significance. This significance is not weighed in diplomas or financial gain but in that of internal satisfaction. You will soon find the significance of reaching your target to oddly be secondary in gratification to the struggles you overcame. Allow yourself to see all struggles that lie ahead, and those hardships you are currently suffering, as temporary. See them as ridges of adversity you overcame when others failed. Be proud of yourself, go confidently, and never forget to appreciate the opportunity, and joy, granted by having a life driven by purpose.

PREFACE

What Is a Psychiatrist?

Most online dictionaries, and even those old compilations of text on parchment called books, would define a psychiatrist as a medical doctor (M.D. or D.O.) who specializes in mental health. Although this definition is an accurate description of the profession, it barely scratches the surface of the ever-encompassing field—a field in its infancy, surrounded by misconception, fear, and even disdain. It is a discipline overshadowed only by virtue of the field's inherent nature of eccentricities.

The complexity of such a field warrants not a sentence, as such, but rather a book's length of information simply to provide historical context, description of principles, and those processes used to extract information. This is all before we have even brushed up on diagnostic criteria, genetic- and substance-related inciting factors, and pharmacology with its vast number of interactions and necessities for specific laboratory monitoring. So far, our explanation, although concise, is a hastily formulated inference, doing little justice to the embodiment and gravity such a specialty deserves. A simple proclamation as such does little to elucidate the many pathological influences and disease states that may present as psychiatric symptoms, complete with unnerving deviations from linear thought, which is itself defined as psychosis. Such deviations often present as the only objective symptom to underlying pathology, possibly representative of the only clue to discovery. It is the function of the psychiatrist to determine the origin of such disorganized cognition as a symptom of illness and how, if any, pathological influences are to be explored before a primary psychiatric diagnosis can be presented as justifiable.

The meticulous psychiatrist, practicing thorough due diligence, spends more time attempting to rule out mental illness than he or she does in diagnosis of primary psychiatric burdens as cause for presenting symptoms. This, in turn, signifies the reason behind the grueling 12-year process and intellectual requirements of undergrad education, medical school, and medical residency. Even better an explanation would be to say it is the psychiatrist who enters the room when other specialties have found their efforts futile. It is the psychiatrist who is not timid, nor afraid, shedding light on what others are unable or unwilling to understand. It is the psychiatrist who becomes the advocate for the patient, one who demands appropriate testing and medical evaluations, being ever astute to defend the patient from having their afflictions succumb to prejudices, their symptoms minimized from unjust stigmas, or their condition cast away and labeled as that of "just psych."

How Does Someone Become a Psychiatrist?

It takes a minimum of twelve years, or 4380 days, to become a psychiatrist. These days are comprised of four years of college, typically with majors in biology or chemistry, followed by four years of medical school studying everything involved or related to human anatomy, physiology, and pathology. Here you deliver babies, perform surgical procedures, dissect, suture, and everything else you could think of regarding the human form. Once this bridge is conquered, one then finds themselves spending another grueling four years in medical residency.

As a resident physician, you spend your first year as an intern responsible for treating patients in a multitude of settings with what would be considered those of "general physician" duties. The last three years of residency are when resident physicians spend the great majority of time in their chosen specialty of study, which for me was psychiatry.

The following stories were taken from those last four years of study during my psychiatric residency in the central valley of California. I have only included those experiences related by some means to psychosis. This was done with the intention of simplification, via structuring the conversation to consist of a single, yet vast, entity of psychiatric illnesses. The symptoms of psychosis are the quintessential examples for all that people fear in psychiatry, and therefore, a great place to begin our journey.

INTRODUCTION

Societal preference is that those with mental health issues be hidden in some remote institution, removed far from society, and isolated from the standard ideal of normalcy. It is most comforting when the "looney bin" is deprived of easily accessible highways that could lead back to civilization. This castle for the mentally condemned should be elegantly encircled by a deep medieval-style moat while still benefitting from modern amenities such as high-voltage fencing and motion-sensing alarms. The mere thought of sharing the same air with "crazy" people for those who are naïve to mental illness is repulsive in the same sense that anything not understood takes on a mysterious, often negative, and fear-invoking association.

Some people with common physical disorders are more than willing to discuss their struggle. They stand sporting the t-shirt of their illness as something to be defined by, a group to be part of, or a souvenir of something they have overcome. This is not true of those people suffering from psychiatric disorders. There are no trophies for overcoming depression, no pink ribbons for mental health awareness, and no t-shirts saying, "Ask me about my schizophrenia."

To avoid the stigma and attention that follows individuals with psychiatric disorders, those suffering from mental illness concede to a life of secrecy, stepping out of the shadows only when they have affixed the mask of a much more passive and traditional exterior. With this façade in place, these individuals never grow to feel adequate or accepted in their entirety, ever-present in the knowledge that others would partake in judgement if they discovered what lies behind the mask. If exposed to the hidden truth, smiles to the front and whispers to the back would become commonplace. This individual, shamed in suffering, is forced to confide in no one. Alone in secrecy, the mind, which is starving for freedom, begins to create dialogue to discover what is wrong instead of realizing what is beautifully unique within. Most don't realize or comprehend that their illness is nothing more than a complication arising from the organ they count on the most. They don't realize that this same organ is actually betraying them—a betrayal from past trauma, insults from substances, synaptic misfiring, or neurotransmitter variations. All this potential insight is hidden by a mind simply trying to make sense of the signals it is receiving.

Some hold the notion of perseverance over all disorders of the brain, using only positive and inspirational talk. This itself is bordering psychotic, as its road of reality has diverged into that of fiction. There is no conquering of mental illness by simply "getting over it." This process of thought is no less probable than the diabetic simply using will and mental strength to overcome a failing pancreas.

No one with any sense of reality would encourage a diabetic patient to forgo treatment with insulin in favor of self-motivating the pancreatic gland, through conviction, to increase its production and secretion of endogenous insulin. There is no simple mantra, diet, or self-help book that will cure Parkinson's disease or stop the insidious progression of Huntington's. These illnesses of the brain are chronic and relentless. They are to be appreciated and respected for their organic origins and their need for appropriate pharmacological interventions.

Any pathological process causing agony requires medical interventions to slow its progression and to provide those afflicted with improvements in quality of life. Abnormalities of the emotional mind, such as jealousy, anger, and disgust, can possibly be improved via constructs of purposeful fixation, yet organic and genetically predisposed psychiatric disorders are conditions of the brain that typically do not conform to commitments of behavioral alterations.

A diagnosis of schizophrenia is no less organic than a diagnosis of dementia, and when the comprehension of this concept is grasped by society as a whole, we will see those with mental illness, not in a light of misunderstanding and judgement, but through eyes of empathic understanding. With this sympathetic tolerance, mental illness will begin to gain acceptance of its origin as chemical, anatomical, or deviations of structure.

There is a mindset that all illnesses should have some quantifiable measurement of testing. Mental illness, aside from its structural etiologies, has no easily appreciable lab values for measurement. This lack of clarity through measurable biological markers in no way discounts the validity of mental illness, for we, as a scientific community, understand very little of the brain's complex processes.

Much of the inner workings of that organ in your skull remain elusive to science fact and largely live in the realm of the hypothetical. Diagnosis of such elusive conditions is left to the artful clinician observing symptoms and allowing interpretation, all to amass hints as to the underlying pathology. In mental illness, determining a diagnosis, and the possible etiology of that diagnosis, is something like searching a vast, darkened auditorium with only a small flashlight. You rarely get to see a lab test or Computed Tomography (CT) scan that lends unequivocal clarity. You never have the chance to flip the switch and illuminate the entire auditorium at once. Instead, you have to painstakingly and methodically piece together clues one at a time. Only then will the light of transparency begin to remove itself from the shadows, and with it, a chance to change the outcome.

DISCLAIMER

In this book, I use the terms "mental health," "mental illness," and "psychiatric illness" all to mean the same thing; that is, a human being suffering with some ailment affecting their emotional state, disrupting their ability to function in society, or impairing their ability to care for themselves properly due to either disorganization or self-harm. I also use the terms "patient," "individual," and "person," all with the intention of simple identification. All terms to me are interchangeable as we are all individuals who at some point in our lives have been a patient.

Great effort has been taken to hold true to the accounts as they happened. Also, all patient-identifying factors have been altered to restrict any chances of infringing on patient confidentiality; yet the stories presented still provide actual portrayals and narratives as they occurred.

This book's purpose is simple: provide an authentic, raw, and unbridled look at psychosis as a symptom as well as an indication of disease states, while elucidating origins and treatments. In this format, I will attempt to educate the reader regarding mental illness as well as provide an inside look at the anguish those stricken by altered reality face. This is not done for our entertainment but with the hope that, through the eyes of a psychiatrist, readers may experience a unique perspective to mental illness. It may be possible that this increased knowledge and awareness of psychiatric disorders may in some small part help to facilitate the dissolution of the stigma surrounding these illnesses.

As a display of respect and empathy for all people that read this book, I feel it warranted to present a warning. The material in this book may be disturbing for some and may trigger previous emotional trauma in cases in which a story relates. The content is at times violent, gruesome, sexual, and containing of strong language. This was not done to shock, but simply to tell the stories as they happened, providing a truth of clarity so that the reader may honestly understand the world of mental illness, the struggles psychiatric patients face, and an insight into the mind of a new physician simply trying to make sense of the pain he sees before him. Don't be afraid of what you don't understand. There is no blanket we can use to cover our eyes from the fears before us. We must provide ourselves with the awareness that knowledge breeds insight and sheds light to the darkness caused by ignorance.

CHAPTER 1

The Zoo

JOSH / KEVIN

"Every life is a play. I am privy to only a single scene in the dramatic essence of a character in turmoil."

For the psychiatric resident physician, the emergency room is an excellent place to study Homo sapiens and how we treat one another. It is not only a place to study others but also the self. This is the first place many of us learn to neglect our empathy, failing to recognize our previously held ideal that medicine is all about helping people in need.

In the ER, we fight to remain guarded against callousness. We fight against internalizing our patients' pain and emotional struggle, instead compartmentalizing each occurrence into a dusty old file in the back of our mind. It is an unchoreographed dance between a vigilant mind, the perception of care, and the struggle to not be the suffering person we see before us. Many of us turn to humor to cope, and some, of course, turn to much more disastrous mechanisms. It is in residency, however, that the physician you learn to become becomes the physician you are forced to live with.

To me, the ER is likened to a zoo, and as such, I would assign everything outside of the hospital as the wild, a place where people frolic without the constraints of captivity, labeled by self-identification aligned with their own ideals. However, in the ER, and more specifically in the psychiatric emergency wing, patients are branded by medical personnel. Staff who typically know little of the human they are dealing with provide classifications for these odd strangers, classifications that are almost entirely based on previous medical records. These records almost always perpetuate misidentifications and amplify the stigma related to mental disorders. We label these captured "bipedals" with medical terms, complete with jargon requiring a doctorate to interpret. These labels aren't simple opinions that are taken lightly. They are permanent stains in the individual's medical record that will follow them for the rest of their life. The record is visible to future physicians, insurance companies, and any employee that walks through the hospital doors.

Analysis of those outside the confines of the ER is trying and laborious; therefore, we wait for the unsuspecting to come to us. We bait them to our zoo with bright-red signs upon a towering building. We even have vehicles with flashing lights and loud sirens to guide the way should they lose their route. Once inside, we trap them in the confines of small spaces. Here we force them to endure the traumatic sounds of people suffering and clinging to life. It all takes place in a brightly lit room, coupled with persistent beeps and overhead voices. Announcements seemingly originate in the sky, calling upon specific individuals for particular tasks.

In the psychiatric ward of the emergency department, we find ourselves faced with the most acute states of mental illness. Psychiatric patients are separated from one another in actual rooms and not the curtain dividers prevalent in most emergency departments. Individual rooms are complemented with a sliding glass door, and each room faces inwards towards the nursing station. This organization allows spectating staff to look upon the developing chaos, each unique in their disorganized presentation.

You couldn't be blamed for this initial reflection when exposed to such a scene. Each patient is suffering in their own fragmented reality, and each experience is as real as the one in the room adjacent and to the one we each are experiencing now. Just as you can feel your hand gliding over the cover of a book, they feel a touch on their shoulder, hear a voice in their ear, or look upon a nonexistent person standing directly before them. Their perceptions may be disturbed, but in the essence of experiences, their hallucinations are their reality. It is a state of awareness no different in subjective reality than the experience you are having now while reading this book.

That being said, how do you know the book in your grasp, or the tablet in your hands, is actually present and not just a visual hallucination? Maybe those around you are simply perceptual disturbances formulated by your mind to make you feel comfortable while you sit in that café alone, sipping your iced chai tea latte.

These patients, labeled as *psychiatric* patients, become restless while awaiting assessment, placement, or discharge. Their confinement to glass rooms reminds me of the fish tanks at the local pet emporium. Instead of fancy guppies and cichlids, we have human subjects. These once free citizens of a larger body of water are forced to swim in circles, not allowed to leave, as we fear certain societal collapse should they escape. Patients are compelled to perform meaningless tricks for a reward, disguised as an emergency room sandwich. Each sandwich is affixed with exactly two pieces of white bread, one slice of mystery meat, and one slice of lettuce. Each sandwich is neatly cut at the appropriate angle to be ingested as triangles. I am sure there is a study that found triangle-shaped sandwiches to be the least offensive of all the sandwich shapes, hence the widespread use of such in emergency rooms around the country.

It's day 2,951, and today will be my first day actually working as a resident. My first rotation just happens to be in the emergency department. After finishing three weeks of monotonous hospital paperwork and orientation lectures on policies, I am ready to get my feet wet, curious if I'll be able to stay afloat. My excitement is only dimmed by the hour of the day. With the current backdrop of rigorous study, one would think my body would have adjusted to little sleep, but my body has remained unconvinced of the importance of arriving at work before the sun rises. Even here, in year nine of training, my body and mind still struggle to adjust to early morning duties. As always, to keep pressing forward, I remind myself that this pain is temporary, while often telling myself that, should I ever have my own medical practice, it won't open till after lunch.

In the first year of residency, you experience firsthand what it's like to be considered a physician. However, a physician in his first year of residency is so low on the totem pole of importance that the medical community would rather refer to them as interns than resident physicians. It's an unnerving feeling to go from medical student to physician overnight. All the safety of being considered inept is stripped away, and it is now expected that you possess a level of experience supposedly garnered by the ring of the midnight bell.

I take a moment to think of the path I have taken to arrive at this moment, either as an introspective look into the struggles I have faced or simply as an excuse to lie in my bed for a longer period of time. For many, there is the road of convenience; for some, there is the road less traveled; but for a few of us, we carve our own path and suffer our deserved fate.

Residency! Holy shit, I made it! I think to myself. I'm not sure why such a realization is internally expressed. Maybe I have found an unused space of air for which to breathe for a moment.

I begin to wonder if I have what it takes to live up to what a physician should be. I think of all of the days I spent as a leaf on the ground under a proverbial tree—a tree that represented all my goals and aspirations. During all the days I spent under those barren branches, I was motivated and appreciative for the opportunity I had been granted, yet I still wished to be picked up by a passing wind and dropped off at the finish.

The measure from undergrad to the completion of medical school totaled 2,920 days. Each day was a day lost with my son. Each day was a day I spent missing the precious moments of his life that I could never recover. Not one day passed that I had not stepped out from under this tree, peering westward, hoping to see the glimmer of home among the flatlands. I would often pray to see a vision of my son running towards me, his hands intermittently rising up as he yells, "Daddy!"

It has been a journey laden with many battles of windstorms attempting to uproot my tree from its source of life. So many days were conquered simply with my head down protecting my resolve from sudden gusts. I have spent so many sleepless nights alone with the only companion being the moon peeking through the branches. Not all days were bad, as there was also a bounty of sunshine, and although the winds remained persistent, they blew west, and west is where I'm headed.

On that final day of medical school, numbered 2,920, I remember waking up to fields of beautiful ever-reaching waves of grass and flowers. I remove my boots, letting this new growth fill the gaps between my toes. As I gather my belongings and begin my journey home, I look back upon the great distance that I have traveled. I began my journey a broke, homeless, discouraged, and hopeless tattooed man with a great history of poor choices and even poorer decisions. Yet, after 2,920 days, I will set my claim to the fields of residency. Still broke, unfortunately, and tattooed, but now a resident physician. It is now time to add sustenance to the roots of knowledge, to allow the insecurities to be covered with healthy flourishing leaves, and to never forget all the foliage lost.

I give one final exhaustive expression of disdain for the alarm clock beside me and gather myself upright from my horizontal state of inertia. Just as I set my eyes to the shower, I receive my first phone call of the day. I nervously look at the time on my phone as well as the clock resting on my nightstand with fear that I have overslept. The call is an urgent consult from the emergency room.

"Hello, Dr. McLaughlin, are you on ER call this morning?" asks the male voice.

"Yes, I am. I'm actually on my way to the hospital now." A partial lie, yet one still based on truth.

"Okay, great. We have a patient we would like you to see as soon as possible."

"Will do. I'll be there shortly," I reply quickly, trying to get off the phone and make good on my previous statement limited in truth. I think to myself that my morning Starbucks routine has just been shattered and beaten. I guess I'll have to start the day suffering from a deficiency of caffeine in my red blood cells. It's a unique form of anemia I have learned to combat when at all possible.

I finally arrive at my expected location and am impressed that I am only mildly late. I find my way down the five flights of stairs of the parking garage and head into the emergency room. It is the time of day when those ending a 12-hour shift are now handing off all the patients from overnight. This continuity aspect of appropriate care is done so pertinent information can be passed on to the next team and each patient can be released from the previous team's responsibility. I check the board and find that, for my patient, it simply states, "Thirty-five-year-old male."

Just as I am about to walk into the patient's room, a nurse grabs my attention and introduces me to the patient's live-in girlfriend. As I approach, I can't help but observe that this woman has two inches on me in height. I introduce myself, shaking her hand as I thank her for being here to help. As we meet in a grasp of introduction, I notice that my hand disappears in the substantial cavity of her much larger hand.

I look behind me to make sure the patient isn't within earshot of our conversation and realign my gaze to the woman before me. I then proceed to give her the information I have, which is nothing but age and sex, hoping she can elaborate while concentrating on the pertinent details.

I have never been particularly attracted to tall, strongly statured women, not so much for lack of chemistry, but mostly due to my own insecurities of having to stand on my tiptoes to kiss my better half. I must admit, however, there is something appealing about a woman who can match you drink for drink and stand beside you in a bar fight as the chairs begin to fly. This isn't the wafer of a woman I am used to. This is the type of woman who would hold the line in battle, with the capability of carrying you to safety if wounded. She is a stunning example of a shield maiden and one I would be willing to stand beside in combat. I stand in her shadow, listening cautiously to the details of her story. Her bright-red hair and matching freckles tell of a probable Scottish ancestry. I could only guess the lineage of warrior blood coursing through her six-foot-two frame.

She breaks the silence of my pause and begins to elaborate on the situation at hand. "He was in the fucking bathroom coughing! I pushed the door open and he was on the floor, gasping for air." She makes the sound of someone with restricted air intake. She also pantomimes the global sign of choking with her hands around her neck as if she was unclear if I could grasp the concept of "gasping for air" without a visible demonstration.

She continues, "I yelled, 'What the hell did you do?' Josh just laid there pointing to the empty cleaning bottles on the floor. I was like, 'Did you drink those?' He just nodded his head. So, I left his dumbass on the floor while I ran to my cell phone to call the police."

She continues, without hesitation, to describe the patient's endorsements of pain and burning in the mouth, throat, and chest. She then details the redness and severe irritation around the lips and oral mucosa. With her cool-headed nature, she had the wherewithal to give the two empty cleaning bottles to EMS (emergency medical services) professionals upon their arrival.

Upon reviewing the bottle's ingredients, it was soon clear that each bottle contained sodium hypochlorite. This dangerous chemical is the primary active ingredient found in bleach and other common household cleaners.

I try to discern some reasoning for his actions. "Do you think he was trying to kill himself?"

"I don't think so, but I have no idea."

I pry further to engage her memory. "So, he has never stated a wish to be dead or wanting to simply end his life?"

She looks up to the ceiling, going through her life's Rolodex of witnessed suicidality. "No, never! Why? Do you think you are going to diagnose him as a 5150?"

I decide to not correct her on proper verbiage and use of the infamous California involuntary hold, the dreaded 5150. The designation of 5150 basically represents a 72-hour, involuntary hold, typically in a mental health hospital. This hold is placed upon individuals that are deemed a danger to themselves, a danger to others, or simply too disorganized because of a mental illness to provide themselves with food, clothing, and shelter. If the patient's symptoms fail to resolve in those three days, then it may be extended to a 5250, with due process, which is an additional 14-day involuntary hold.

"Well, I need to figure out what's going on first and then we will decide as a team what is best for Josh. My main priority is to keep him safe."

Dissatisfied with the rapid decompensation in the absence of clear inciting factors, I attempt to discover clues leading to such a severe act. I press his girlfriend for more information. In doing so, I learn of a chronic history of psychosis for which he is prescribed psychiatric medications. She relays that during med-compliance, Josh is "pretty normal," but that about six weeks prior he refused to take his medications any longer "because he felt cured."

Next, I make my way to a computer and start sifting through the piles of data regarding current and previous visits to our hospital. I look for medical clearance to assure he has had a full work-up. The hospital I'm in usually does a great job with "psych patients," as the emergency docs, for the most part, are caring and compassionate to the struggle of psychiatric illness. Each psychiatric patient must first be evaluated for medical issues and subsequent medical clearance before we, the psychiatrists, will even attempt to communicate with the patient to formulate a speculative diagnosis and plan. It's a way of checks and balances—a little annoyance of habit that serves the purpose of being an agent for those who cannot fend for themselves.

This requirement of full medical clearance entails all the appropriate testing you would provide to any other non-psych patient. We as psychiatrists can then be assured that our patients are treated as equals, and for a moment, the world appears fair and just. Without such medical clearance, many patients with psychiatric history have their medical issues discarded as products of their mental illness. My request is simple: "If you want them out of your ER, then first do your damn job and work them up as you would any other patient. Then, and only then, will I facilitate a plan for treatment or discharge."

From his electronic medical record, I see Josh has a psychiatric history with no less than seven previous psychiatric hospitalizations over the last five years. It appears the general consensus is that of auditory hallucinations, paranoia, and thought disorganization, all in the context of intermittent meth use with sporadic positive urine drug screens.

His medical history, along with the collateral information provided, paints a picture indicative of someone suffering from schizophrenia. With such a diagnosis comes the cold hard facts that without his medications, his ability to determine reality will likely become residual, with psychosis overwhelming the majority of his perception of the world around him. Many times, patients with schizophrenia wish to stop their medications, not only because the extended lack of psychosis makes them believe they are cured, but also as a relief from the sedation these medications can cause. Unfortunately, as seen with Josh, the honeymoon period of increased energy and alertness often comes with the price of divorce from reality.

I can see that he has been appropriately screened for adverse effects of his "drink of choice," and I am satisfied that he received a thorough evaluation. His assessment comprised of airway management, endoscopy, chest x-ray, EKG, urine drug screen, and a battery of blood tests, just to name a few. Luckily, he was found to be without esophageal, or other, perforations, and had been monitored over the recent hours for stabilization. Thankfully, the patient was found immediately post-ingestion and transferred quickly to the emergency department.

Now it's up to me to figure out how we got here. I take a moment to gather my thoughts as I glance towards his room, trying not to get caught up in the ordeals of the rooms flanking him. Both rooms on either side of him contain patients who are waving through the glass for someone to assist them. The glass is adorned with their foreheads pressed upon it in some coordinated effort to garner attention. The chaotic nature of the psychiatric emergency department can be a nightmare for anyone with deficits in sustained attention. However, I remain focused and enter what appears the calmer of the three options.

"Good morning, Josh. My name is Dr. McLaughlin and I'm a psychiatric resident. The emergency docs asked me to come say hello and see if there was anything I could do to help you."

"If you could fix the air, that would be great." His quick rebuttal gives me some insight into the delusions to come.

"Tell me, what is it about the air that concerns you?"

"It's full of toxins and metal particles. The government puts things in the air to make us sick and to control us."

I attempt to clarify this segment of delusion so I can make an effort to understand the area of cerebral misalignment he is suffering from. "So, what was your remedy for the toxins and metal particles that you feel you have been inhaling?"

"I drank fucking bleach! Hell, if that won't work, what will?"

Upon assessment, I quickly see the concerns of the primary medical team. It is very clear that, while the patient may be medically uneventful, he is far from psychiatric stability.

I notice right away a multitude of visible tattoos. He appears to have a general disregard for socially acceptable restraints, displayed by the numerous piercings in his lips, eyebrows, and nasal septum. I know immediately that I will have to relax my style to earn his trust.

I notice his speech is low in volume. I gather this is due to irritation and swelling, but rather than assume, I simply ask. "You seem to be speaking quietly. Is it because of the injury to your throat?" It's then I get a glimpse into the true depth of his paranoia.

"They're always fucking listening!" he responds in an expressive whisper. The volume of his speech is even more dramatically decreased than the statement beforehand, yet still loud enough for anyone to hear. His inability to quietly utter his thoughts and perceptions is likened to a child loudly whispering as they underestimate the acuity of the human cochlea. He points skyward as to indicate a greater power, extraterrestrials, or maybe satellites. Thankfully, he continues to divulge the secrets hidden inside his own mind.

"They can hear everything I say through my teeth."

"How do they do that?" I ask.

"The metal fillings in your teeth, man! The government listens to everything we say. They are documenting my life."

"Wow, man, that sounds horrible!" I reply, creating a common enemy and earning trust. "How does that work? How do they listen through the fillings?"

"Satellites. It's all satellites. They have a satellite that follows me everywhere I go. They have a frequency that taps into the metal fillings. You know what else? I think this all has to do with the Illuminati. They must have put a microchip inside me to control me. My pastor said they anointed me with the oil of madness."

"Well, it sounds as though you have a lot on your plate, and it must be quite the burden to bear. Tell me what I can do to help you through this situation." I'm bargaining as to provide a platform for him to display some semblance of sanity.

"Get me the fuck outta here! That would be helpful."

"Okay, I understand you are dealing with a lot of shit, but you need to do me a favor."

"Sure, man, whatever it takes."

"I need you to take a little vacation over to the mental health hospital."

"Ssshhhiiittt, man, I don't want to go back there," he replies with all the same phonological processes of a Southern drawl.

"I understand. I wouldn't want to go there either. But for safety reasons, if I let you walk out of this hospital and you die or complete the next suicide attempt, I would be stuck doing a shit ton of paperwork. Not to mention I'll probably get fired and have to go to trucking school." I witness him laughing yet at the same time wincing in pain.

I continue: "You won't be there long, but I truly believe it will be helpful." I end with a smile and a chuckle and he reciprocates, displaying a reactive mood. "Plus, your girlfriend is going to beat your ass for you almost killing yourself. It's best to hide at the mental health hospital for a while until she cools down."

Shaking his head in disgust, he is trying not to laugh again and trigger more pain. "That's true. Fine. I'll go. You know, you're not like any doctor I ever met."

"Well, I'll take that as a compliment," I reply, shaking his hand and giving him one last smile. I walk out of the room accepting this ordeal as a win for the patient. He will most likely not suffer from any residual physical complications due to the swift medical care he received.

I believe Josh will fare well in his stay at the mental health hospital. They will restart his medications, make adjustments as needed, and steer him back to reality, all while keeping him safe from contaminated air, pesky satellites, and the ever-present Illuminati.

The day continues on and remains more or less uneventful. With a quick glance behind me, I see it's nearing 9pm, which signifies only three more hours until the conclusion of my shift. Of course, on day one, another resident called in sick and I am stuck covering half of their shift as well as my own.

It has been an odd day in the emergency room, and although I love every moment of it, I would be willing to appreciate the comfort of my own bed just as well.

I find myself, once again, sitting and waiting for whatever comes through the triage door while trying not to think about the heaviness of my eyelids. I quickly find myself lost inside my own head and adrift into absence. I should go find another source of caffeine but decide against it in favor of a mental vacation. I don't think anyone will notice my cognitive truancy. The nurse to the right of me is texting on her phone, and the doctor supervising me is examining his ex-wife's Facebook page, and neither could care less about the catatonic gaze I'm developing. Awoken from my stillness by the buzz of a call bell, I sit up too quickly, making the annoying creak of the computer chair come alive while gaining the uncomfortable gaze of each colleague flanking me. Finding myself back in the present time, I clear my throat and shake my head in concurring disapproval of the chair.

No sooner did I gather myself than I hear my name being shouted. "Hey, McLaughlin, we got one for you," someone in triage yells out, followed with a giggle. It was in medical school when I learned to greatly fear the giggle from triage.

I get up reluctantly, praying that I don't have to do any rectal exams—what I call "the ER handshake." It is yet another favorite for staff to pass along to the unsuspecting medical student, and during those four years, I certainly embarked on my fair share of human awkwardness between two strangers that only such a procedure can produce. You would be surprised, but a higher-than-expected percentage of people that come to the ER get a finger up their ass, fancily called a rectal hemoccult test. If you have complaints of blood in your stool, blood in your spit, dark stools, vaginal bleeding, weakness, anemia, or any number of other conditions, plan on having a stranger's finger in an unwelcomed place. Personally, I think "ER handshake" has a better ring than "rectal hemoccult test."

I also hope I don't have to withdraw any further misplaced items from unintended orifices for the rest of my life, fingers crossed. I will never look upon a large, rounded, glass, holiday-scented, Yankee candle the same way after one particularly nasty ER experience. Thankfully the case coming from triage today has nothing to do with rectums or misplaced candles.

Just as the bellow from triage arrives, the door to the ER opens and the parade makes its way through the door. The entourage includes two ladies with clipboards—I'm guessing they are social workers of some type—one police officer who does not look the least bit amused, and one child, all being followed by two more police officers. *Wait, where is the patient?* Patients don't typically walk in with clipboards and they usually, and I stress *usually*, don't come dressed as police officers. That leaves the child. *Three officers for one child? Well, time to put on my serious and concerned face and get to work.* I step forward and introduce myself. Just as I begin to mutter my normal introduction, I'm swiftly interrupted.

"We got a twelve-year-old boy here charged with bringing a weapon to school and making threats," the first officer says to me in an authoritarian voice, implying with his tone that this was serious but also not so serious as to require the necessary paperwork he knows undoubtedly lies ahead for him. I bend down to greet our miniature convict. "I'm Resident Doctor Mclaughlin. What's your name?"

"Kevin," he replies quietly with eyes fixed to the ground.

"Nice to meet you, Kevin. You can call me Patrick. Sound like a deal?"

Kevin says nothing but does give effort to unexcitedly nod his head in agreeance.

"Okay, everyone, please follow me." They shadow me as I guide them to the secluded psychiatric area of the emergency department.

In hospitals, and in the general public for that matter, psychiatric illness is not understood or appreciated as an organic process. It's this misunderstanding that leads to a negative stigma. Mental illness is feared, and rather than try to understand its origins and constructs, it's stuffed away into the shadows. I lead the convoy to an area in the back corner, reserved solely for patients suffering from mental illness. I picture the architect drawing up plans for the building saying to himself, *I better put those psychiatric patients off to the side and away from normal folk. We can't have their crazy infecting the rest of the patients. A mere scratch from a crazy person could infect the victim with the same disorder of lunacy.*

We find our place and begin deliberation. The court of jaded opinion is now open, and the prosecution has the floor for opening statements. I get the rundown from the officer and then from the social workers. Both stories sound eerily similar except I prefer the latter as it was in a more relaxed and sweet voice without the pungent inflection. No sooner is the prosecution about to rest than in comes the parents.

A solid parental interview can be the most important part of determining the psychiatric wellness of a child. Any and all collateral information—meaning that which is not given by the patient—can be of great importance. By talking to the parents, you get a glimpse into what this child has had the opportunity, or the burden, of living with. Not to mention, many psychiatric illnesses have a genetic component, so this is a great way to see what genetic material mom and dad may have so graciously passed on to their children.

Clinical assessment for a child of this age with reported psychosis is tricky. The list of possible etiologies is vast, and all must be ruled out prior to being labeled a primary psychiatric disorder. Something that also must be considered is the rarity of legitimate childhood-onset schizophrenia.

Testing includes magnetic resonance imaging (MRI) of the brain to rule out central nervous tumors and to look for any gray matter loss that may be seen in those with childhood-onset schizophrenia. Blood tests are done to test for complete blood counts, glucose, and electrolytes, and to assess liver, kidney, and thyroid functions. Urine and serum toxicology is also warranted to rule out substance-induced psychosis. Concurrently, we have to rule out a quite extensive differential, which is a list of all possible causes and contributing factors such as a seizure disorder, encephalitis, chromosomal abnormalities, autoimmune disorders, metabolic disorders, and even heavy metal poisoning. Even if all tests return "within normal limits," we still need to rule out autism spectrum disorder, major depressive disorder, bipolar disorder with psychotic features, and post-traumatic stress disorder (PTSD), just to name a few.

Psychiatry has gone through a reconstruction of core beliefs, and the days of psychoanalysis as the sole treatment has passed. We now understand that psychiatric illness is no different from disorders in other organs, and we appreciate this newfound biological orientation. We now treat patients with a mixture of psychotherapy and focused-psychopharmacology, all backed by evidenced-based research.

I feel the next step in psychiatry should be the re-designation of disorders based on their pathophysiology as done in other specialties of medicine. For example, hypothyroidism isn't called "tired-and-cold disorder," and congestive heart failure isn't commonly referred to as "shortness-of-breath disease." The typical classifications in medicine are based on pathophysiological causes, or derivations, rather than symptoms. Therefore, major depressive disorder could be referred to as hypo-serotonin syndrome and may be labeled as such someday—that is, if the serotonin-hypothesis is proven to be valid. As computational neuroscience dissects causes of mental disorder, the names of these diseases should change to fit such causes. This will in turn provide more validity for the diagnosis as being biological in origin.

I greet Kevin's parents as they approach, offering each a handshake and an introduction of my title and role. Kevin's mother introduces herself first. "Hello, Dr. McLaughlin,

I'm Karen." Karen looks to be the quintessential soccer mom with a handbag as large as a suitcase and short brown hair that can be easily done in times of rushing children to school. I can see she has been persistently crying today as her mascara is all but gone, except for small, faint streaks mapping the travel of her tears.

Kevin's father is still wearing garage attire due to an obvious rush to get to the hospital straight from work. His nametag reads *Kyle*, and underneath that is a label that says *Fred's Automotive.*

As I begin to interview Kevin's parents, his mother starts in right away and is visibly concerned. I listen carefully as she describes months of torment, not from her son, but from her feelings of despair. Her despair is the kind that you only hear from a mother who truly loves her child but feels she is failing in some way.

She describes how Kevin has been talking about seeing some figure and about how he is paranoid someone, or something, is after him. She describes multiple occasions when she could hear her son talking to someone while alone in his room. The speech she describes is not simply that of someone bored and occupying their mind with self-talk but that of a bona fide two-person interaction.

She talks about their multiple counseling sessions and family meetings, all while I quietly listen for clues. She talks about different psychologists and psychiatrists and how each one, in her mind, has failed to show the willingness to truly help her son, or at the very least failed to appreciate his illness. As she reaches into her purse to show me a letter her son had written in his diary, a large folder falls out.

I can see the contents of the folder immediately and recognize this folder is filled with drawings. I quickly ask to see it and meticulously look over the pictures as the mother continues.

At this point, I hear nothing the mother says as I am fixated on what I'm holding. The pictures have all the signs and skill one would typically see in the drawings of a 12-year-old boy, yet something about these drawings is unusual and odd. It's not so much what each depiction is missing but what is present. No matter what the scenery, no matter what the context, each drawing has a figure. This figure is the same in all the drawings. Not similar, but exactly the same. It's in the window of his house, at the foot of his bed, behind him on the swing—it is ever-present in drawing after drawing.

I look at the pictures and get a weird lump in my throat. I feel the hair on my arms stand up ever so slightly. This figure sparks some innate fear in me. I can't express the feeling except to say it had a familiarity that went straight to my unconscious. I feel immediately sad and concerned for this boy. The figure is dark, ominous, and cold, without eyes or expression. It is without form but just human enough to be recognizable. To me, this figure encompasses everything that is evil.

I gather myself and look at the mother while holding one of his drawings up for comment. I can tell in her eyes we are not thinking the same thing. I look to the father, standing beside his wife, and I scrutinize his expression, but yet again I am met with no reciprocation of the emotion I am feeling. I then take another drawing and hold it up to the father to get some sort of human reaction.

I always find it strange when a parent discounts the claims of a child, attributing them to be merely a product of an over-active imagination. This is especially disturbing when the claims refer to odd content, strange beliefs, or threatening situations. I understand a child's mind is active in imagination and the developing brain is taking in sensory information trying to assemble justification to avert danger and to fulfill curiosity. I understand sometimes this leads to the spilling over of imaginary concepts or perceptions, but to not listen and inspect such statements from a child is a huge injustice and a blatant disregard to subjective validity.

We have all seen those movies where the child is being tormented by an entity, and as soon as the parent opens the door, the entity retreats back to the dark and the child attempts to explain the reason for their scream. Even though the child is white-knuckled and in obvious distress, the parent discounts the possibility of anything but some innate fear of the dark, reducing worry to nothing but childhood misperception of stimuli. Without even a hint of inquisition, the parent sternly states, "Go to bed!" They retreat, closing the door behind them, subjecting the child to face the monster alone with only a blanket to shield them from their adversary. Now, of course, most movies of this type will progress in this same fashion until the entity makes itself known to the parent. There is nothing more satisfying than watching the parents in their "ah ha" moment as you feel vindication on the part of the child. However, are we any better than those parents as we discount every remark or explanation that does not fit in our preformed pattern of thought?

"Yeah, he's always talking about that guy, this boogeyman or whatever you call it," the father says, as he shakes his head in disappointment.

I ask him quietly, "Do you believe him?"

"What?" his father asks, obviously determined to not allow my whisper to stay as such.

"Do you believe him?" I sternly ask although still in a reserved volume.

"Well, yeah, I believe he thinks he sees this imaginary guy," Kevin's father responds.

I can tell by his answer that we are light years away in thought of possible derivation of this entity. It is at this point that I should have ceased this line of questioning, but now I am curious. For some reason, this feels like more, but I can't place my finger on what. I try one more Hail Mary pass, hoping to hit the end zone.

"Are you religious?" I ask Kevin's father.

"Well, if you mean, like, do we go to a church, then no, we're not." His response has a hint of frustration and confusion.

I step back graciously and pepper in some medical talk, explaining the typical medical history and onset of symptoms to hopefully appease his perplexed state. I step back to lick my wounds from the lack of insight into Kevin's ordeal so far. It's then when I notice the soot from the father's auto shop has nicely adorned his clothing with a dark veil of oil and grease. His face and hair both contain the same tinged remnants, giving his overall silhouette a homogenous darker shade. One could say if he was to present at the edge of a bed, he could be mistaken for the dark, ominous figure so prevalent in Kevin's life.

Dare I traverse this possible incestuous path? I think it's unfounded at this time, but it will remain a grain of sand in my vision with its irritable discomfort reminding me of its presence.

I turn my attention to what transpired today. Kevin's parents are more than willing to voice their disapproval of their son being suspended from school. I again ask for the details of the incident without the bias subliminal insertions.

Kevin's mother decides to take the lead commentator role. "Well, apparently, he sent a love letter to a girl he likes, who happens to be in the same class. The note said something like, 'No one believes me, but I know you do. He is trying to kill us, but I won't let him hurt you. I brought a knife to protect you.' I guess the girl showed the teacher and, sure enough, he did have a kitchen knife in his backpack." Her details of the incident provide me with additional insight into Kevin's psyche, and I thank her for her input.

In this current time of school massacres, bringing any weapon to school is not something the educational community takes lightly, nor should they. No one could fault their decision of suspension. However, from his perspective, he was trying to protect himself from a threat that was real, maybe only to him, but still subjectively authentic.

Our kids grow up watching violent tv shows, programs where turtles transform into ninjas and defend themselves, and their best friend April, from a gang of henchman led by a man called the Shredder. How do you think these green heroes defend themselves and protect the helpless April? Well, with punches to the face, kicks to the groin, and sharp-bladed weaponry. How hard is it to surmise that, for a pre-teen, this wielding of a knife was appropriate, especially when defending his life or that of the ones he cares for? Blunt trauma and evisceration are what our children grow up on, yet we expect them to sit quietly while reading Chomsky and sipping elderberry tea. I am sorry, but you cannot hope for peaches when you plant an apple tree.

I decide it's time to interview the man of the hour. I find Kevin sitting in the hallway, strangely quiet and free of any of the unintended psychomotor agitations people usually display during times of stress. There is no constant looking around, no hands tapping, no restless legs, no changing of positions. He just stares ahead at the blank wall before him.

Kevin appears to be your average, husky, 12-year-old boy. He is free of gothic paraphernalia; I doubt he owns an "f-the-world" t-shirt. He's just a normal-looking child from a hard-working family. Both biological parents are actually married to one another, which is rare, and the father is actually present and still in his life. That's certainly a positive foundation for a child. For all I know, they have a cottage-style home with a white picket fence and a Labrador Retriever named Spot. Yet here we are.

I ask Kevin to follow me into an empty interview room with an examination table adorning the middle. I leave the door propped open ever so slightly so that we may have a private conversation and still allow others to pass by to view our session. Kevin sits up on the aging exam table adorned in brown faux leather, his feet hanging over the side. Kevin is inattentive and initially dismisses the symptoms as "just playing." He seems like a bright child from the way he carries himself, much too young to be so stoic. It is most likely this same intelligence that is telling him this situation has become too intense, and for survival, his mind is convincing him to deny all symptoms.

Fortunately for me, what he can't control are his eyes. They give him away and relieve any question of validity, as he intentionally tries not to look over my right shoulder. It's not what he is looking at but what he is avoiding that gives me all the data I need. He avoids gazing over my right shoulder as if there is an abnormally bright light shining towards him, scorching his eyes with every deliberate look. This doesn't keep him from quick glimpses of fear. I witness his eyes dart to the left, checking to see if what behind me still remains.

This behavior is referred to as responding to internal stimuli. Stimuli that we normally respond to is that of external stimuli, or the presence of objects or sounds based in reality. This differs from internally generated stimuli, which is created in the brain and is only truly present in the brain. This betraying brain generates misguided impulses, leading the mind to display images towards a witnessed stimulus that is of no realistic validity. The room is void of all persons and objects, other than the two of us and the table; therefore, he is not misinterpreting a fixed object in the room, commonly referred to as an illusion. What he sees is coming from inside him, inside his mind.

For Kevin, this betrayal is interpreted as paranoia and fear, with that manifestation of fear obviously standing behind me. Throughout the interview, he remains guarded and laughs at none of my comical references, which could be indicative of his negative affect or the unlikely theory that I'm just not funny. His affect remains flat, which basically means his range of displayed emotions is nonexistent. He presents with no change in facial expression throughout the interview, which is again another distressing sign.

"Do you have friends at school?" I ask.

Kevin simply shakes his head.

"Okay, then who do you eat lunch with?" I ask, trying to catch him in some sort of incongruent statement.

He simply replies, "I eat lunch alone."

"That's okay. I actually prefer to eat alone as well," I remark, trying to normalize the daily dose of lunch loneliness we commonly share. "Kevin, tell me why you took a knife to school."

"I don't know," he responds while shrugging his shoulders.

"Kevin, I want to help you. You are in a safe place, but if you don't talk to me, I cannot help you."

He takes a deep breath and reluctantly begins to tell me something. "The dark man." He stops and removes his gaze from my direction back to the floor.

"What about the dark man? Tell me about him."

"He wants to hurt . . ." Kevin begins to lower his guard and just as quickly stops mid-sentence with no recovery back to the subject at hand. We call this *thought blocking*. Thought blocking is a psychiatric phenomenon where someone's speech ceases after they have begun to talk. It is typically a disruption of speech from a patient who has been interrupted by auditory hallucinations. Imagine being in the middle of a conversation and someone runs up and starts talking in your ear. Your first inclination is to stop talking and listen to what is so important that the intruder felt it was necessary to barge in upon your current conversation.

"Did someone tell you not to talk to me?" I ask, partly already knowing the answer.

Kevin discretely nods his head. "Yes."

As I ask question after question, it is like pulling teeth. Kevin gives me very little other than one- or two-syllable answers. I fear pushing too far within our brief first encounter may be more deleterious than beneficial. It becomes obvious, rather quickly, that Kevin is in a different world. Kevin's only interaction with me is through a small window, and unfortunately, it's a window that Kevin has closed shut and drawn the shade over.

The clinical severity, impact on development, and poor prognosis of childhood-onset schizophrenia is very real. Positive symptoms, such as hallucinations, are necessary for the diagnosis in children, as imaginary friends should cease to exist by the age of six. Symptoms of psychosis, which basically equates to any condition affecting perception leading to a removed sense of reality, are altogether rare in healthy children.

Childhood-onset schizophrenia is an extraordinarily rare illness that is poorly understood, yet when present, appears to maliciously continue through adulthood. Not to mention, diagnosing a child with schizophrenia has profound effects on the treatment course, including the potential for neglecting another disorder, as the symptoms of psychosis often become the primary focus.

Fortunately, I never had the chance to burden Kevin's future with such a diagnosis. Unfortunately, I also missed the chance to follow the progression of his illness, its treatment, and the opportunity to play a part in his hopeful recovery. A children's psychiatric hospital about 90 minutes away had an open bed, and my hospital ER was all too happy to send him there. Emergency room physicians are pressured by hospital management to get patients out of the ER as soon as possible.

The transfer of Kevin was inevitable, and a children's psychiatric hospital is more adept at handling such a detailed and severe child psychiatric case as Kevin's warrants and deserves. That is the thing about the ER; you only get to see the patients for a short time. You learn their story, you find a position of worry in your heart for them, and then, just as quickly as they fell into your life, they are gone. Transferred to another hospital, discharged, or admitted to the hospital floor. All these areas are considered out of range for the psychiatric resident working in the ER.

The thought of spiritual influence scares me many times more than other influences of the brain. In the spirit of Kevin, I wonder about the religious associations of mental illness and where the line of religion and biological disease blur, and where they find clear divergence. All religions are based on faith and the ability to believe while buying into foundational, religious stories of wonderment. Are all these religious stories built upon psychotic features? Do miracles, possessions, or feats of spiritual influence occur today, or are such preserved only in our history? Although much of our populous today hold religious convictions, such incidents that would have once been held as wondrous are now discounted, and such inference to anything other than biological is less than welcomed in our age of cell phones and internet dating.

Physicians are no different than non-medical folks in that our brains' first inclination discounts every remark or explanation that doesn't fit our preformed pattern of thought. When did scientific facts lead us to believe that limited conclusive proof equals impossibility?

I once had a professor who took me aside and scolded me for what he called dualism. He used to say I was too intelligent to believe in such farces as ghosts, demons, voices from the sky, men who walk on water, and those that rise from the dead. He would ask me that if I was so certain I had a soul, then to tell him its location. He would also interrogate my plan of afterlife, baiting me to show him the location of this so-called heaven. He had his data, and I had my faith, so we never did see eye to eye. I guess I'm just destined to be an idiot of faith in his eyes. Which of us is correct? I guess we will both have to wait for our own mortality to determine the validity of each other's positions.

I still see Kevin sometimes, not in person, but in the adults I see with schizophrenia. Sometimes I wish that what was plaguing Kevin was spiritual; then maybe I could just call upon a priest to perform an exorcism, and move on. Unfortunately for Kevin, this is most likely not the case, and the demon he will face will be lifelong and ever-present inside his mind. For now, it remains an unexplained case of innocence interrupted.

CHAPTER 2

The Zoo Part 2

JUSTIN / REBECCA

"Cocaine is God's way of saying you're making too much money."
—Robin Williams

It's day 3,002 and I continue to settle into the groove of this new hospital. Today I find myself with a new crew of unsuspecting coworkers. I scan the area and overhear conversations. I quickly measure experience and perceived intelligence, not in judgement but simply as procedure. I quickly surmise which nurse I can go to if I have a question. I learned in medical school that a physician is only as good as his nurse, and as a resident physician, I would often call on their experience and knowledge for maneuvering my way through the hospital. A great nurse will also catch your mistakes and, with a whisper, save you some measure of pride. Most do not realize, but nurses run the hospital. They are the front lines of patient care. The nurses' acumen is often the difference between life and death in acute and traumatic situations. These same nurses, however, can make your life absolute hell. I pride myself on being extra kind to nurses, not just as a measure of ass-kissing, but also from a place of respect. The resident physician is a visitor, and each area of the hospital is someone else's home. I was taught at a young age that before you walk inside, you best knock first, ask to enter, and take off your shoes by the door.

The evening starts off rather quickly. The first patient I encounter has already been cleared for discharge; however, he remains seated calmly in his room. I see the patient seated at the edge of his hospital bed, facing the glass sliding door. It's not odd that he remains in the emergency department; what is peculiar is what he is wearing. Although it's not my place to judge others, in this case, I am somewhat amused by what is before me.

The patient appears to be in his late 20s or early 30s based on body habitus alone. He is wearing regalia of the comic book character Spiderman in what appears to be a rather intricate costume. Both hands and feet are covered in the red and blue signature colors provided by the two-piece design.

What makes the ensemble particularly disturbing is that the open area for the face is on the back of his head. The hooded part of the costume, instead of resting appropriately in the rear, is pulled tightly over his face. It appears to be thin enough for oxygen transfer and basic visualization of shapes and fluctuations in light, but tight enough to see his nose flattened in an upward direction. It looks more like a guy with pantyhose over his head to disguise his identity on his way to a bank robbery than a superhero I would call for assistance in a time of need. I stop for a second to take the entire scene in just long enough to think, "I don't want to know," and since he has already been cleared for discharge, I walk onward to the intake area to see what is in store for me tonight.

Before I know it, I find myself attending to a patient who has been waiting for psychiatric clearance for a good part of the evening. I advance to his room with only the knowledge that he is a male in his late 20s who was brought in by family because of a traumatic blow to the head. Apparently, it was only after he was triaged that it became apparent that this patient may be better served with a psychiatry consult prior to discharge.

I enter the room and provide the usual introduction and shaking of his hand. He has deep black hair, which appears dyed as his eyebrows and overall complexion point to a more subtle color. His long black strands of hair are styled in a circa 1980's mohawk. The sides and back of his head are shaved. He looks at me with a wide-eyed gaze that's even more pronounced by the addition of eyeliner carefully drawn onto the upper and lower eyelids. There is a faint yet visible outline of darkness around both the upper and lower lips, most likely also the result of an overzealous lipliner pencil.

I start with a generic form of questioning to figure out why Vince, the goth character from *Portlandia*, is sitting before me. This is a memory aid I use for future recall of the patient. This is what my mentor in medical school would call a "pink hat." While on inpatient psychiatric rotation, with 16 to 20 patients under our care, he would say, "Find the pink hat in each patient to help you remember them." It can be a physical trait or something comical, but it really does help to remember the intricacies of each patient. When you have ten patients with psychosis, you can't just say, "You know, [insert name], the guy with psychosis." However, if you were to say, "You know, [insert name], the 'shit thrower,'" you would instantly think of the individual that has been hurling his feces and doing so rather frequently. With this indexed tab of a "pink hat," you remember their name and everything pertinent to their case. These memory keys of association and connection are a lifesaver when seeing a high number of unique individuals each week. I stop fixating on the Portlandia character and find myself back at work.

"So, Justin, tell me a little bit about why you are here."

"I got hit in the head!" He says this without gesturing to the injured area, as most do in cases where they are describing an area of the body.

"Okay, well, who hit you?"

"I was in my bathroom when some guy came up from behind and hit me in the back of the head." He shows little expression as he speaks, incongruent with such an attack.

"Did this person use any type of weapon?" I ask, as I slowly draw my eyes to the back of his head, straining to see the severity of injury.

I witness no less than eight vertical mattress sutures—different, and slightly more complicated, than the simple interrupted stitch pattern I typically use. Of course, as a psychiatric resident, individuals are less than excited to hear that I'll be operating on their precious skin. Most, rightfully, prefer the surgical or emergency residents for such a task. Therefore, my ability to find willing candidates to allow me to practice has dwindled over the years. I actually do enjoy the process of suturing lacerations and other wounds and had quite a bit of experience doing so in my medical school rotations. I imagine what draws me to liking such a procedure so far removed from my specialty is its simplicity. The procedure ends in a finished product that is acutely appreciated in adding completeness to an individual. The human is a strange animal that focuses solely on such separations of skin. The wish for totality and integrity that the integumentary system provides is not only comforting but also highly precious in maintaining our freedom from all that is around us. I digress and continue with the conversation at hand.

"Yeah, he hit me with a pipe," he responds.

"Do you know the person who hit you?" I ask.

"I don't know who he was, but he had the body of a horse and up top he was a man."

"Wait! So, let me see if I understand you. The guy that hit you was half man and half horse?" I am feeling more confused than I should. I nod my head to appear concerned while withholding the smile that is dying to emerge.

"Yeah," he answers while also nodding his head. This is not so much as to add further validity to his story but simply, and unknowingly, mimicking my behaviors.

"You mean a centaur?" I ask for further clarification.

"Yeah. A centaur!" he exclaims as if he had been searching for the word for hours.

Of course, at this point, any normal physician would order a toxicology screen and walk out until results arrived. I did nothing of the sort; in fact, my only responses were those in line with my creed to "always give the patient the benefit of the doubt before discarding their story of events."

"Why would a centaur need to use pipe?" I ask without the feeling of silliness that should accompany such a question.

At this point, I'm not sure if I was just provoking further thought in him or if I was truly curious. I mean, horses must weigh at the very least a thousand pounds, so even just half a horse with a human torso has got to be somewhere in the range of six-hundred pounds. You would think an intruder that size wouldn't need to use a weapon to overcome a mere human. I continue to rationalize the situation and find discrepancies in his story, not because of the innate presence of a mythical creature but because of his chosen weapon.

I truly enjoy stories such as these. It's as if you are given a glimpse into the brain's capability for creativity and uniqueness. These obscure depictions of reality also allow a glimpse into the brain's capacity for betrayal. Listening closely, you can almost hear the mind struggling to decipher the misguided code of neuronal firings, looking for meaning through justification—a justification often provided through elaborate and mystical interpretations.

I continue our montage for a short time, which is now more entertaining than informative, and I run the gamut of questioning regarding danger to self and others. I lead into some questions of orientation and other basic neurological assessments, which he, surprisingly, does rather well with. Justin has no complaint of headache, nausea, or vomiting. He displays no gait instability, and his pupillary reactivity is normal. I still plan to order a CT scan to rule out any intracranial abnormalities.

For now, however, I give our tortured human character a much-needed respite and a temporary pass on further questioning. I feel any further recollection about the incident, although interesting, will most certainly contain very little usable information. Although he vehemently denies any substance or alcohol use recently, the dilation of his pupils suggests otherwise. Therefore, urine toxicology prior to moving forward will also be of utmost importance.

As I finish up with Justin, I start to think for some reason about my job and how intriguing this brain of ours is. It is an organ that can fully alter our compass, misguiding our course and steering us away from reality. The cardiologist works on the heart, which is basically a four-chambered mechanical pump. The psychiatrist works on an organ with billions of neural connections, an organ that is capable of calculating mathematical equations, writing, and painting. It's an organ that is even capable of falling in love—through specific release of neurotransmitters that are rewarding and construed as love by the willing mind, of course.

It's an organ that derives your future while containing the self and all its past experiences; an organ that ultimately determines your personality and how you experience the world; an organ that the mind is tasked with interpreting, allowing miscalculations of neuronal connections to manifest in an endless form of perceptual disturbances. All the while, the heart is still just a pump.

Most like to say psychiatry is the study of the mind, not the brain, which is less than inaccurate and borders on foolishness. You cannot separate the brain from the mind. You cannot separate emotions or behavior from the pathological functions of the brain. Our emotional aspects are sometimes the only outward manifestations of our intricate brain, creating a window into the function of all those billions of neuronal connections. There is no mind and brain separation; it is one conglomerate. It's a never-ending dance of cause and effect, with those effects manipulating future cause. The drugs we use as psychiatrists don't just work on some mysterious fluffy substance inside the skull, they work on that big ol' brain of yours and its oversized neocortex.

The brain is a beautiful blank canvas of complex possibilities whereas the mind paints its own impression onto this canvas. Sometimes the mind is beautifully organized, offering the onlooker a straightforward impression of the world around them. Well-positioned trees gently interrupt the landscape, all brought together by a life-giving river just over the hill and past the quaint farmhouse. Other times the mind is a meth-addicted abstract artist who aggressively throws cans of paint on the canvas with no rhyme or reason for its placement. Here the artist basically states his impressionistic concept of, "Fuck it, you try to figure it out!" This certainly doesn't display the formatted thought of conceptualization of life to canvas; however, it does give rise to an interesting set of symptoms that you and the patient are forced to carefully sift through.

I walk out of the room, still reflecting on matters of scientific marvel, when I am nearly run over by a fast-moving stretcher. The EMT steering this speedboat through the ER yells out a quick, "Sorry, Doc!"

I see the EMT settle into the psychiatric intake area and I slowly walk over to the patient. She is still bound to her vessel of transport by two "safety-belts" crossing both upper and lower limbs.

I settle into the stool, some feet away, and listen intently for clues. The nurse is presented with a flurry of information as the EMT gives an enthusiastic and in-depth report of the new addition to our dysfunctional family. Reading from his small flip-up notepad, he rattles off all the information he gathered on scene. His voice is loud and his cadence rapid, stopping only for small breaths of fresh air as he attempts to impress the crowd around him.

"We got a twenty-seven-year-old female here, brought in by ambulance after her father called 911. She has no medical history, and dispatch said the father reported his daughter has been 'acting strange' lately." Air quotes are provided by the EMT for dramatic effect or to disagree with the minimization of her symptoms by the father. "Patient is afebrile with an oxygen saturation of ninety-eight on room air and appears hemodynamically stable."

I gather my thoughts and give the patient a quick once-over as I introduce myself, dragging out the words of my introduction to allow myself further time for inspection. The top of her skull catches my attention, with not one but multiple deep gouges littering my field of view. It looks as though someone has taken a melon scooper to the top of her head and made a human-fruit salad. The large wounds are obvious against the background of her pale, white, clean-shaven head.

While attempting to determine the cause of such injuries, I notice the wounds are linear and roughly the width of a human fingernail. I look down to her hands, which remain in soft restraints and tied rather close to the side of the stretcher. She struggles to gain movement without progress, intermittently appearing frustrated when her efforts towards independence are ineffective.

Her fingernails appear jagged, with dark sediment remaining under each of the nails. The remnants of sediment appear less like soil and more like that of dried blood. Her hands are providing a pattern indicative of someone who has spent the better part of a night willfully peeling the flesh from their own head.

"May I ask your name?"

"Yeah, I'm Rebecca."

"Nice to meet you, Rebecca. My name is Dr. McLaughlin. I'm a resident physician here at the hospital. Now, I'm just going to come out and ask. What made you shave your hair off?" I ask this not only to break the ice but out of curiosity.

"What hair?" she answers, looking perplexed.

"Exactly!" I give a short giggle, obviously thinking I'm funnier than I truly am. I pretend she answers with some coy answer regarding the utility and cleanliness of not having to tend to such strands of time-sucking maintenance. I continue to have the conversation with myself as she remains utterly confused as to its relevance to her. I think to myself; *I should do the same. Shit, I would save a lot of time each morning.*

I ask frankly, "What the hell happened to the top of your head?"

"I need to get out of here as soon as possible. I have a booty-shaking contest tonight in L.A. I need to win! I need the money, and I'm not going to let that bitch Bambi win again."

"Okay, well, I will certainly do my best to help you get out of here as soon as possible." I choose not to respond to the booty-shaking comment. It could be misconstrued as non-professional if I was to inquire, even though I'm curious as to the validity of her claim. She doesn't appear to have the body of a booty-shaking champion, yet who am I to judge. For all I know, I could have the queen of the booty-shaking world before me and not even realize it.

I attempt to garner another explanation for the wounds on her head. "Rebecca, can you tell me how you got these injuries on your head? Did someone hurt you?"

Dammit! I think to myself. I just executed one of my most despised question formulation strategies by asking her two questions in succession. There are two reasons I never do this. First, because it's useless, and second, because it's useless. When you give a patient a barrage of questions in succession, they will often only answer the last question. This creates a situation where you need to ask each question separately again to be sure what answer goes with which question. It is one of my biggest pet peeves and something I pride myself in not doing.

"Oh, that's nothing, it's fine." She responds as if I had asked about her opinion on the temperature in the room.

"Well, it certainly doesn't look like nothing. Can you try to at least tell me what happened?"

"That's not real; that's movie make-up. Someone put it on me as a joke when I fell asleep."

"What do you think is movie make-up? I'm confused." I'm trying to find some sense of clarity to the situation.

She attempts to calm my concern. "Those cuts on my head aren't real cuts, they're just movie make-up."

"Do you have any idea who did this to you? I mean, who do you think put the movie make-up on your head?"

"Probably people that make movies," she replies. "It's not real. It's fake. Get my hands out of these straps and I'll show you it's fake."

Well, she is correct, as I'm guessing people who make movies have access to movie make-up, but I'm not so certain that the use of her hands will change my opinion regarding the bloody, oozing holes in her head—holes indicative of large chunks of meat gone missing.

I realize that using a mirror to show her the wounds upon the top of her head may be difficult, especially in her current position. Instead, I move towards a different route for the potential of insight and in the spirit of patient-centered care; I decide to temporarily remove her "shackles."

"Okay, I'll release your right hand so you can feel what I'm talking about. You have to promise me, no funny shit, or I'll have to put the straps back on your wrist."

"Okay, I promise," she quickly responds.

I slowly release the Velcro to the right wrist as I motion with my eyes to the security guard perched just outside the door to move in closer. Once released, I take her hand and help fit each one of her blood-stained fingers into a sterile glove. With my own gloved hand, I guide her slowly, showing her the depth of the injuries, all as I talk her through the process.

"Okay, Rebecca, do you feel this?" I slowly glide her fingers over untouched skin. "Okay, now can you feel this?" I allow her fingertips to glide over one of the wounds, allowing her finger to appreciate the depth of injury.

"Yeah, that's not real. See!" She pokes her index finger straight into one of the wound channels as if she was being fitted for a custom bowling ball.

"Please don't do that!" I say rather loudly and sternly, quickly realizing the lack of wisdom and experience in my thought process.

"But it doesn't hurt. It's not real. I'm not crazy. Do you think I'm crazy?"

"No, I don't think you're crazy," I reply.

"So, you believe me?"

"Well . . . I believe you have four to five particularly deep wounds on your head that will need to be addressed, and then you and I can chat more. For now, I just want you to relax and I want you to stop picking at the damn movie make-up until we get a chance to clean it off for you."

"I knew you wouldn't believe me. You're just like everyone else."

"It's not that I don't believe you. I'm just a resident physician, so I have to find an attending, who is my boss, and show him the make-up on your head before we can do anything else. You understand what I'm saying?"

"Yeah," she reluctantly answers. "I just want to go home."

"Okay, I'll see what I can do," I reply, knowing damn well she is certainly not returning home anytime soon. I am guessing there is some chronicity to her disorganization, as her delusions appear quite fixed. Pending collateral from family and, of course, medical clearance, she most likely will be heading to our inpatient mental health hospital until we can get her psychiatrically stable. Before stepping out, I motion the guard to follow me. Once we step a few feet out of the room, I turn and ask him to keep an eye on the patient. "If she goes digging into her head again, please restrain her right hand back into the soft restraints or call me and I'll come do it."

I head to the other side of the ER, the place without all the screaming, and find the emergency medicine resident on duty. I relay that the female patient in room 3C is cleared for medical evaluation as I have gone out of order of typical protocol simply because of timing and proximity to the new arrival. I confirm his plan is not to catch-and-release until I get the psychiatric assessment team down for a 5150 evaluation. He agrees, and I head straight to the waiting lounge with hopes of finding Rebecca's father and, with his help, shed some light into what the hell is going on.

Rebecca's father jumps out of his seat when I call his daughter's name, and I take him into the adjacent conference room so we can have a chance to talk in private. He confirms that Rebecca has been off her psychiatric medications, more specifically risperidone, a second-generation antipsychotic, for nearly 60 days.

Her father elaborates that over that time, Rebecca has suffered from multiple acute exacerbations of her chronic schizophrenia, each time leading to admission to the inpatient mental health hospital. He describes the content of her psychosis to be those of auditory hallucinations via the birds outside her window. Apparently, she spends a good part of her afternoons conversing, and yelling, at the birds outside her home. Sometimes she can be found chasing these same birds outside, running in circles around the home, all the while screaming profanities at these winged instigators. Rebecca's father remarks that his daughter claims the birds speak to her in a derogatory and almost taunting manner, and do so purposefully, just to frustrate her.

He continues, stating that most evenings she is heard in her room, conversing with herself and laughing inappropriately, often during all hours of the night. He relays the fear that if he falls asleep too soundly that his daughter may do something to inadvertently harm herself. This worry has plagued his own restorative sleep, which is obvious by the look of defeat upon his face. I do my best to assure him that we will do everything we can to help.

He appears to be a caring father that enjoys his daughter's presence in the home, but he is also grateful to hear of my plan for involuntary hold and transfer to the mental health hospital. He understands it's the safest place for his daughter to recover in her current disorganized state. He looks hopeful as we part yet overwhelmed with exhaustion. I'm sure a few days of respite care is more than deserved.

Due to Rebecca's current exacerbation of psychosis and delusions leading to self-harm, I request the psychiatric assessment team to evaluate her for a 5150 hold with transfer to the mental health hospital. There, she will be placed in a locked unit where she can be monitored for safety. Her medications will be restarted, replaced, or adjusted until at which time she reaches a level of baseline functioning—a level of function where she can reliably demonstrate safety, free of any further, impending harm to herself.

Later that evening, I find myself searching for sustenance and end up in the hospital cafeteria. Shredded pork sandwiches are on the menu tonight, covered in some red enchilada sauce, or manufactured chemical equivalent. As I start to indulge in my carnivorous offering, I get a flashback of Rebecca. I recall, unfortunately with great detail, the separation of skin from her underlying flesh. The sight of this red-tinged meat appears eerily similar to the brilliant red shade found only on that of a freshly severed wound. I oddly associate the separation of her scalp in shape and color with that of my shredded pork entrée. I quickly push the tray away and to the edge of the table as this thought has, at the moment, separated me from my appetite.

CHAPTER 3

The General

FERNANDO

"Sometimes two people can say nothing,
and everything, at the same time."

As our brains struggle to automatize our actions, it's difficult for a psychiatrist, or any physician for that matter, to see repeated symptoms consistently and to not become desensitized to the slight variation in the presentations. We must struggle to stay vigilant in searching for the subtleties. Our patients deserve better than automated processes in exchange for individual treatment that is unique as the patient themselves. Sometimes, these unique treatments encompass treating those in strange locations with strange tactics.

It's day 3,029, and today I get to meet with Fernando, or as how I think of him, *The General.* Ever since I met him, the General has become one of my favorite patients. This is strange because we never actually speak to each other, at least not in a verbal language that we both understand. With a Spanish translator, day after day, I call on the General. He has now been in the mental health hospital for over a week, and managerial staff is pushing me to discharge him. He suffers from schizophrenia; however, his personality, both kind and friendly, blinds others to the underlying suffering, or at least the functional impairment, his disorder generates.

When a schizophrenic patient doesn't appear to be foaming at the mouth, most assume his condition is improved and appropriate for discharge. Schizophrenia, as a fundamental construct, has a plethora of functional impairments, with some not so clearly visible. It is not easy to look at someone and determine that they are too paranoid to seek food or shelter. The lack of willingness to engage in activities of daily living isn't always displayed in screams of psychotic dialogue. In contrast, conceptual lack of self-care, or present paranoia steering one from such care, can be highly dangerous. Aside from the media's perception, schizophrenia can present as a quiet and flat outwardly appearance. This state of tranquility can actually be an accumulation of internal perceptual disturbances, disorganization of thought and speech, and a significant failure of functioning in life as well as in social interactions.

For Fernando, his disorganization is one of duty to country. He suffers from a delusion that he is a general in the Mexican army receiving messages, in the form of military instructions, from television commercials. This situation, when people believe a neutral event such as a television commercial is actually a personal message of instructions, is referred to as a delusion of reference.

Delusional or not, I enjoy finding him every morning in front of the television in the recreational room. Without deviation from his routine, he is present daily, at 8am, standing at attention and awaiting further instruction. He is often found responding to television commercials with such intensity and purpose that occasionally I wonder if he is truly receiving messages.

I still remember the first time I witnessed his reception of orders from the television. It was first thing in the morning, and I had just arrived at work. Hoping to get a jump start on my day, I snuck over to the locked unit to start my assessments, knowing I'd likely have to wake most of my patients up from their medication-induced slumber. As soon as I opened the door, I heard repeatedly the utterance of, "Plata o plomo? Plata o plomo?" This was followed by an obvious definitive answer as the phrase ceased and this gentleman standing uncomfortably close to the television in the day room began to nod his head in agreeance. With the cessation of information being provided from this television, the gentleman stepped backwards, abruptly locked his feet together, and performed a perfect military salute. After I was done spectating in marvel, I procured the assistance of a translator and went to work.

"Hello, Fernando. My name is Dr. McLaughlin." Obviously, this was not in the beautiful cadence or sentence structure of his own native tongue. He turned abruptly in our direction and blessed us with a genuine smile. While pleasant, this initial conversation would set the stage for many conversations that led to zero insight into his illness. He would consistently deny all psychiatric symptoms in his joyful state without any malicious intent subdued behind the smile. He was genuine and his care was simple; maybe that's why I appreciated seeing him first every morning. It's hard not to smile when someone greets you with genuine kindness followed by a military salute.

Every day after that, he greeted us with the same warm smile and good morning wishes, in Spanish of course, as well as a proper military display of respect.

We were never able to procure much historical data about him, and there was no family to gather the collateral from. He was alone, and because of such, his chances for success status post discharge were minimal.

According to the 5150, the General was found roaming the streets, responding to internal stimuli, and flagging down civilians for much-needed logistical information regarding his current military engagement. Where this delusion began and how it became so well-seated in his psyche will remain a mystery.

Delusions are like herpes: difficult to treat and never fully removed. They linger, lying in wait, only to spring forward as visible as a cold sore on your upper lip. A delusion by definition is a fixed, false belief. These unshakeable beliefs are not easily eradicated even when the person is presented with evidence to the contrary. People with delusional disorder typically have one or more delusions. These delusions, apart from the inherent impact of such beliefs, usually do not markedly impair the individual either socially or occupationally. People with delusional disorder can also experience hallucinations; however, these perceptual disturbances are not prominent and are usually related to the delusional theme of the person.

These delusions can be one of a multitude of flavors, some highly palatable and forgiving while others downright frightening. Now, as a caveat, one cannot qualify for the diagnosis of delusional disorder if their delusions are secondary to overall symptomology of schizophrenia. As we all know by now, or will soon learn, those with schizophrenia suffer severe impairment in daily functioning as well as a multitude of other symptoms.

The General is unfortunately suffering from something greater than a belief that he has simply served time in the military. His delusions are not the case of delusional disorder but likely of a more ominous condition. His symptoms are severe and dramatically impair his overall functioning. His auditory hallucinations and delusions of reference are prominent, all indicating a diagnosis of schizophrenia.

The General continued to respond to the television, and we were never able to break his delusion. Since he was able to complete activities of daily living and was not a danger to himself or others, we had to discharge him to a homeless shelter. This was unfortunate, as I would have liked to hold him longer so we could devise a discharge plan with greater services, as I feared he would decompensate without them.

Over the next two months, I saw the General out in public multiple times. The General was everywhere. I would see him walking down the sidewalk and marching through parking lots, always smiling and always expressing his opinion with someone no one else could see.

On day 3,106, I find myself nearly late to work again. I'm heading back to the mental health hospital for my night call shift. Rushing home to grab dinner took longer than expected due to traffic. I decide to take the freeway back to work; sure, it's longer in overall mileage, but at 5:50 pm, it seems like the smarter route. As I move speedily down the freeway, safely balancing a water bottle between my legs as I eat a bowl of my usual dinner (chicken and rice), I see something, no! some*one*, on the side of the freeway. I spot a man standing on the side of the freeway yelling at cars as they pass. This man is approximately thirty years old, Hispanic, and appears to be wearing only pants, with no shirt or shoes.

"Oh shit! That's the General," I say out loud.

I quickly pull my car to the side of the freeway and call 911. The 911 operator is amazed by my detailed knowledge of this random person. I exit my car and walk down the side of the freeway towards him. I remember having a newfound appreciation for the speed at which we travel in our vehicles, something only standing on the side of a busy freeway can provide.

I walk about 15 feet from the General and begin to yell his name.

"Fernando! Fernando!"

He turns around once but doesn't seem to identify me outside of the hospital. I continue to garner no attention from him, even as I risk looking psychotic myself. I step further onto the freeway, ever closer to traffic, yelling his name. He, too, increasingly advances into the roadway, obviously frustrated with the cars and their lack of respect for his military position. I have difficulty determining if Fernando is yelling at the people in the cars or the cars themselves, but I assume the latter. It must be infuriating to evoke zero response from these passing hunks of steel, all potential soldiers in his army of delusional purpose. I watch with ever-increasing worry.

Just then I see a small SUV swerve quickly to avoid the man in its path, the mirror of the car barely missing his torso. The operator of the vehicle provided his middle finger as a gesture of goodbye, honking his horn as he accelerated away. The time spent with his hands on the horn seemed excessive, not indicative of a warning but more of a disgruntled expression of anger. I can only speculate, but maybe this anger was for the sanctity of life he nearly obliterated or maybe such reaction was derived from the driver realizing that the near-fatal miss would have considerably complicated his day should they have made contact. I would have rather he stopped and helped me guide a fellow human from danger, but he obviously had more important matters to attend to.

I finally see my fill of near misses and sternly yell, "el General."

He stops immediately and does an abrupt about-face. I respectfully salute him, and he, in turn, salutes back. I then gesture with my arm to sit down next to me, as if I was welcoming someone into my home. I direct his attention away from certain death, via any one of the 3,000-pound hammers traveling at 70 mph. Fortunately, he is temporarily brought out of his reality to an alternative view of a less dangerous truth. It is not such an authentic truth that most would consider reality, but for us, this is enough.

For a moment, we sit by the freeway occasionally shaking our heads at one another in agreement of something unknown and unsaid. We understand nothing of each other's past, or even language, but with simple head nods, we have created a dissertation paper on international understanding. I sit next to him, my car hazards blinking faintly in my right eye as my car patiently waits a good 30 to 50 yards down the freeway.

I had never before enjoyed the simple pleasure of sitting under a freeway overpass, and surprisingly, I found it quite calming. The passing of the cars plays a beautiful consistency of white noise with the comforting roar of passing combustion engines. The smell of gas and rubber mixed with oil give the familiar scent of some of my favorite times, reminding me of the days spent working on my motorcycle and the hours of testing my resolve at ridiculous speeds.

In the distance, I see a flurry of lights slowly closing in on our sanctuary. I'm almost saddened by their quick response, as it has interrupted our tranquility. I slowly stand up and he does the same. I offer my hand and we shake. He gives me a final look as the cavalry gets closer and a closing nod of approval. I do the same. He turns around to walk away and stops cold, he does a crisp about-face and provides me with what seems to be the perfect salute. It is a salute with so many possible meanings, but one that seemed to say, "Thank you." I reciprocate, and just like that, he is gone.

I'm not sure what the secret ingredient is, but some patients just make you care about them. I'm not certain what has guided my positive countertransference towards the General. Maybe he reminds me of an old friend. Maybe there is a reason my eyes swell with faint tears when I transfer our experience to the computer screen, often not appreciating the gravity of a situation until stepping back and placing the recollection of emotions into words. It's possible the General simply reminds me of the frailty we are all composed of, hidden beneath the surface yet easily uprooted pending different situations or different histories. Maybe our inner self can see innocence, an innocence that is universal, above gender, above ethnicity, and even above our spoken language.

CHAPTER 4

The Sociopath

ALLEN

"The world is a dangerous place to live;
not because of the people who are evil, but because
of the people who don't do anything about it."
—Albert Einstein

Day 3,049 starts off like any other. I find it amazing how quickly I have become desensitized to the wicked ways of man. We have the innate capability for destruction and seeing this in unscrupulous forms daily would make anyone struggle to hold their positive core beliefs—beliefs we should each hold in order to realize that these perpetrators of evil are not the majority but the exception. The fact that these human exceptions have become the majority you see on any given day does not change the balance outside the walls of the hospital. All medical professionals have to face similar events, each having to choose which patients to hold internal and close to the heart, and which ones to file in the dusty bookshelf of memories in our mind. In this dust, they lay suppressed from cognitive inspection. We can only hope the stories of these patients never fall from the shelf, interjecting their reflections into our actions, ruffling our sense of self.

A late-night patient from prison always makes for an interesting interaction; unfortunately, this patient provides me with doubt in the human race. As I search for the prisoner among the many possible rooms, I'm led by the clanking of his chains as they leave a sharp blow to the ear with each inflection of his voice. He is a man who is accustomed to speaking with hand gestures in concordance with his mouth, but with chains now affixed to his appendages, any speech provides a rattle of metal on metal. He is a talkative man, no doubt, and from a distance I can imagine that, with each word, life is slowly draining from the correctional officer tasked with babysitting him. I always wonder if prisoner transport is a coveted assignment for the correctional officer charged with the task. Maybe the simple freedom from the prison setting, even for a short time, is enough to warrant jealousy in those correctional officers confined within the walls of their respective chosen career paths.

I locate my patient and request the invitation to enter from the officer in the corner of the room. I take my seat across from the patient in the orange jumpsuit. He introduces himself as Allen, and I reciprocate an introduction amid normal pleasantries. Allen makes no waste of the audience provided and proceeds to afford me a story of wrongful conviction and plights of innocence. He provides me with many examples of injustices within the legal system. These educational nuggets are followed by attempts to convince me that he was not in his right state of mind when he committed whatever acts led to this moment. I struggle to find the reason for his visit to the emergency room. Every one of my attempts at redirection is discarded as he precedes to lead away from the topics of my question. A prime example of a tangential thought process is when someone will respond in a matter related to the question at first, then abruptly veer off down a new road of thought, never actually answering the initial question.

I finally realize this session will continue until the next ice age unless I take control. "Allen!" He abruptly stops talking, and I finally have his attention. "Allen, I need you to tell me why you're here in this emergency room."

Without context or an appropriate transition, he emerges from his temporary silence. "I need you to evaluate me for insanity. She told me she was going to take my children away from me."

"Who told you this?"

"My wife. We were married for fourteen years, and out of the blue, she told me she wanted a divorce. She said that I'd never see my kids again. I blacked out, Doc. I don't even remember what happened. When I woke up, she was gone, and I have no recollection of what happened. It's not fair; I wasn't in control."

"Okay, let's slow down for a moment. Was your wife harmed?" I ask cautiously.

"Yeah, she's dead."

"And I'm guessing you're claiming to recall no details of her death?"

"Yeah, I don't remember any of it. I had a break of insanity."

"Can you tell me what you saw when you regained a sense of self? I mean, when you came to, what happened?"

"Well, when I snapped out of it, I saw blood everywhere, so I called 911." He continues to display an affect of incongruency, as this story should create a severe sense of sadness, or at the very least some hint of emotional turmoil. Instead, he tells the story as if it happened to someone else's wife for whom he had no passionate connection.

"Allen, I'm really trying to understand what happened. Let's explore this from a different viewpoint. What did the police find when they came to your home?"

"They found my wife in the kitchen. Apparently, someone killed her with a knife and then used my axe, which, mind you, was all the way in the garage. Someone then used the axe to chop off her head. They found her head in the pool. Now they are trying to convict me of murder when I don't even remember doing it. How is that fair?"

My thoughts become silenced. I try to pull myself from the dense mist inside my brain, as such a story creates a sense of murkiness in the mind. It is an act so vile that it is incomprehensible, and the brain struggles to forget what it has just heard. My mind continues to feel muddled and

I struggle to not picture the scene described. My mind betrays me, and my vivid imagination wins over. It begins to take control. I can all but picture the gruesomeness of the scene described. I picture a loving wife and mother just trying to find safety from a man she no longer trusts. I speculate there were signs of his capabilities before this act that his wife must have decoded—a mother's intuition to save her children from the monster she had conceived them with. I picture her poor lifeless body in a beautiful, yellow sundress adorned with sunflowers, her shoes still affixed as her intentions were to flee. All of it is lying in a puddle of blood. Then a trail of droplets begins to lead the eyes out the rear sliding glass door and into the backyard. The water of the pool is no longer a beautiful blue but instead stained a reddish hue.

I look to the man across from me, scooting my chair back as to not allow the evil within him to taint my clothing. "Do you feel any remorse for what you have done?" I ask. I'm not sure if I was curious about his viewpoint or further trying to cement my belief in his profound level of sociopathy. Regardless, the answer he provides will be of little use as, in this setting, it is not my place to determine insanity in regard to a crime. My only job is to make sure he is not currently harboring acute intent to harm himself or someone else.

"Well, yeah. I'm sorry she's dead, but it's not my fault, my brain just snapped. I blacked out in a fit of rage. How can you be convicted for something you don't remember? Plus, she said she was going to take away my kids. Now, look, I'm the one who has to endure prison, possibly for the rest of my life as I try to regain my freedom. This is all over something that was not my fault. She got away easy, she's dead. I'm the one that has to suffer."

Not often do I discount a patient's point of view, but today, I did. It took all my strength to bury deep the anger I was feeling. I needed to be free of bias and judgement to provide appropriate medical care. Rather than get into a moral debate with a sociopath incarnate, I simply fulfill my obligation and provide a thorough mental health evaluation. I make my recommendations and then abruptly walk out. There is very little one can do to change the mind of an individual devoid of responsibility or guilt. I find it best to simply stay clear whenever possible.

These are the stories that drive psychiatrists, lawyers, and correctional officers to lack of sleep and inner frustration. It can be hard to see the world with the same rose-colored glasses after the knowledge of such evil. We have to struggle to suppress the evil from infesting our own minds. I find it helpful to grow the belief that most people are good. For stories such as Allen's, I have a very distinct shelf far away from conscious thought where he and his story will fit nicely, resting in a slumber surrounded by other perpetrators of malicious deeds that will all soon be covered in grimy soot. They are forgotten deep within the mind as to keep it hidden and overlooked in favor of memories much more pleasing to the palate—memories more indicative of what I believe to encompass the true possibility of the human condition.

CHAPTER 5

Walking Dead

JOHN "ABRAHAM"

"Families are the compass that guides us.
They are the inspiration to reach great heights,
and our comfort when we occasionally falter."
—Brad Henry

On day 3,190, I find myself in the inpatient mental health hospital. I'm still a first-year resident, which is code for fresh meat to some of the more violent patients. While my exterior is somewhat solid, I have yet to build up the callous interior that so many seasoned physicians carry. I remain somewhat malleable and very much open to suggestions.

I gather my patient assignments for the day when one of the assessment logs catches my eye. It has been flagged with a sticky note and reads, "Warning: High Risk." These assessment logs are not where one would go to find detailed patient historical information. It is, however, a good source for a quick "heads-ups" regarding patients that need to be seen and their reasons for admission or consult. These logs are officially known as psychiatric assessment team logs, also known as the P.A.T. logs.

The benefit of the P.A.T. logs is that they are concise regarding reasons for admission, providing just enough content to start the conversation. The negative of these logs is that they are too brief. More times than not these rushed appraisals of mental illness fail to capture the true essence of the person or the instigations leading up to the patient's downfall. However, the logs are *meant* to be brief and to deal solely with the surface-level symptoms that are present. Each is typically written as a legal nugget, justifying involuntary holds or other services rendered.

In typical daily fashion, I head to the unit just before patients are served breakfast. I scan my badge to gain access to the outer door and then again through another. I travel down the hallway, past offices of administration and those reserved for residents. I reach the unit and again scan my badge, going through the two inpatient doors and finally arriving on the ward. I am greeted with a rather quiet scene as most patients are still slumbering in their beds, hopefully each dreaming of ocean waves and fields encompassing a kaleidoscope of wildflowers. I begin to negotiate the scene before me, searching for a man fitting the description of "Warning: High Risk." I laugh to myself, knowing that the most dangerous person on this ward is probably me, the resident physician—the physician-in-training who must appear confident yet truly knows just enough to be hazardous to unsuspecting patients.

One wrong medication cocktail, oversight of previous allergies, or drug interaction with non-psychiatric medications given concurrently, and the patient is a corpse. At the very least, the patient could suffer from worsening psychosis, increased suicidal ideations, stiffness, rigidity, permanent tardive dyskinesia, or a potentially deadly adverse event in the form of serotonin syndrome or neuroleptic malignant syndrome. If the patient is over 65, forget it. My medications can cause increased falls, organ failure, and sudden death. The only patient that others should "approach with caution" is the "patient" with the white coat and the keys to the building.

Many a time, while in training, we prescribe a certain medication to a patient simply on the basis that it's one that we have never used before. We are attempting to garner more experience with it while using the patient's specific illness as a guide. Of course, there are studies, and often FDA-approvals, with each medication in said cases, but until you prescribe it, you will never feel comfortable in dealing with its adverse effects or realize its potential for psychiatric re-alignment.

I unexpectedly spot a man that looks like the stunt-double for Abraham from the television show *The Walking Dead*. He appears to be in his mid-forties, Caucasian male, and about 6'2", with pink skin and red hair that is matched with toned facial hair. He even adorns the distinct handlebar-style mustache so fittingly worn by the character in the zombie saga. He is pacing back and forth in the hallway just outside the recreation room, occasionally lifting his head to the ceiling, cupping both hands to each side of his head, and letting out a grunt of frustration. I utter his given legal name in an inflexible tone, yet all I hear is Abraham. He quickly gives a turn of the head in my direction, then pivots his body towards me. He walks towards me in the suggested motion of a crushed man. His arms swing with an over-reaching arc, likened to that of a pissed-off teenager, as if to say, "Damn, now I must face my shit!" This look is something that is not as unique as one would think. It's the typical look I get from patients who realize that they are about to discuss their deepest of days. Often, I am the second or even third person for whom they have recounted their timeline of misery, which makes the complaint of body language all the more prevalent.

I am not one that is often mistaken for a physician. I remember the first time I walked onto the floor of the ICU, which was during a medical school rotation. I was wearing scrubs, which because of their short sleeves displayed my tattoos, all while sporting a healthy beard. It was at this time an attending of mine approached me and, in front of the rest of the students and staff, remarked, "You look like a convict who accosted a real physician and took his clothes. Looking at you makes me feel like checking all the closets, knowing I'll find a poor, unsuspecting doctor tied up in just his skivvies, with a gag in his mouth."

We all had a good laugh, although inside I couldn't help but feel foolish. Unfortunately, I didn't have the insight, nor proper judgement, to pursue such a career early in life, and because of such, my alternate life path is visible in my frame, stature, and plethora of artistic representations. It's nothing but dumb luck that those same tattoos actually serve me well in my chosen specialty. I now have the ability to dress for the patient and adjust to the situation. I attempt to give each and every patient the psychiatrist they need, at that time in space, regardless of the psychiatrist they want.

For Abraham, I stand tall with the sleeves of my collared dress shirt rolled up, brandishing our commonalities.

I give him the typical introduction and quickly say, "Let's chat."

I open the interview room door, which is actually just behind me and adjacent to the nurse's station. I invite him into the room and motion for him to sit in the chair opposite the desk. I wedge the door open, for sake of protocol, with the short grey-plastic trash can next to the door. I take my seat on the side of the desk closest to the door. I do this, just as I do for all patients, because it's policy, knowing damn well that if the patient turns on me, I'll never make it out fast enough nor would I ever try to run; it's just not in me. If the situation escalates, it will just be the two of us in this eight-by-eight-foot cell, and I accept the task of attempting to subdue this man without inflicting any harm or delivering any blows, while at the same time, trying to survive the blows I will assuredly receive. I don't trouble myself with such worries, as I see this as part of being a psychiatrist. Now for most psychiatrists, I suggest a "panic button," as well as a safe exit plan. Call it foolish male pride or just over-confidence, but I have no need for exit plans and I wouldn't be caught dead wearing a "panic" button, often offensively referred to by unrefined residents such as myself as a "rape whistle."

What they don't realize is that the panic button gives no specific location once activated. In fact, security has no idea which staff member alerted this silent security system. Therefore, it could be anywhere from five to thirty minutes before they rule everyone else out and find you. By that time, some large psychiatric patient, dead set on harming you, has already knocked you unconscious and had his way with you. Maybe the foolish are the ones carrying the whistle, hoping it will save their ass in time of need. Maybe they should be carrying the knowledge to manipulate proper angles, visualize cues to impending violence, and establish proper situation control, rather than relying on a magic button to save their ass.

"Before we get started, I have a very serious question to ask, and I want you to be honest with me," I say, preparing him for what comes next.

"Of course, Doc," he replies, awaiting some shrewdly comprehensive question.

"Okay, good. Now, my question is actually a two-parter. One, do you watch *The Walking Dead*? And two, does anyone ever say you look like Abraham from that show?"

He laughs in relief, all the tension sucked out the small crack in the door created by the trash can door-wedge. "Hell yeah! I get that all the time."

"Okay, so from now on I'm going to call you Abraham. Calling you John seems sacrilegious to a man that looks exactly like Abraham. Is that cool?"

"Fuck yeah, man."

That's usually what I attempt to do. Start strong to set an underlying tone of authority and then at some point, early in the interview, pepper in some comedic relief to get the patient to relax, all the while, displaying empathy, understanding, and the four techniques of active listening: paraphrase, summarize, clarify, and reflect. The key, in my opinion, is to be, or at least appear to be, nonjudgmental. It's about relinquishing judgment, even to the point where you relinquish your own preconceived perception of reality. Instead of judging, I commit to a mental, and verbal, understanding of my patient's most disturbing thoughts or actions. If a patient connects with you as a psychiatrist, understands his or her fall from the ledge of functionality, and feels validated in their struggle and suffering, they will entrust you with holding the ladder as they climb out of the pit.

We move on to explore Abraham's most recent stressors, and he relays the burden of life, unemployment, and financial struggle that has pushed him over the proverbial edge of sanity. I was taken back by his willingness to open up so quickly and completely to me during our initial conversation. He was obviously a man looking for help and willing to leave his pride outside the door.

"I was going to hurt her, Doc!" Struggling to look me in the eyes, he is clearly ashamed of what he just confided in me.

"Who were you going to hurt?" I ask.

"My daughter." He takes a deep breath to assist in holding back tears. "We were driving down the freeway and this voice inside my head was telling me to hurt her. I didn't want to. I love my baby girl. I was afraid I would actually do it, so I pulled over and made her get out of the car. On the fucking freeway, Doc! Who the fuck does that?"

"A man that loves his daughter does that." I pause to let that sink in. "Your daughter was in danger from voices you were having trouble controlling, so you did the only thing you could to protect her. That takes a lot of strength, man. Now you're here to get help and to get your mind right. I'm going to make sure that happens."

We continue to talk, and the more I learn, the more a picture of schizoaffective disorder takes shape. This disorder uniquely affects people, in that, in addition to delusions, hallucinations, and disorganized thought, they also suffer symptoms of a mood episode such as major depressive or mania. It is often confused with schizophrenia, major depressive disorder with psychotic features, or bipolar disorder with psychotic features. Schizoaffective disorder separates itself, first, by the display of chronic symptoms of psychosis, second, during times of concurrent depressive and manic episodes, and third, in times without such mood states. Often patients suffering from this disorder receive the most complicated of medication cocktails to stabilize mood, treat depression, and contain the psychosis. This is not to say people with schizophrenia are never depressed;

however, the severity of such mood states is often more pronounced in schizoaffective disorder.

We dive further into his psychiatric history and I uncover previous episodes of suicide attempts, drug abuse, and persistent psychosis.

He does his best, in his current state, to describe the progression of his illness as a young man to the exacerbation of symptoms he currently suffers from. "I just have so much noise in my head, it's hard to focus on what exactly you want to hear."

"Well, just tell me whatever comes to mind. No pressure." I console him, trying to relay some sense of relaxation.

"I get these voices, both male and female, in my head. They tell me fucked up things about myself and tell me to hurt others. Sometimes the voices almost sound like other people's conversations, like I'm picking up transmissions from people's phones. I know that sounds crazy, but that's just how I think. Honestly, most of the time I don't know who or what the fuck I am."

I have so much I want to say at this point, but I hold my tongue and become the person he needs right now: the doctor that just listens.

We then explore his past, leading us to a seaside tale of suffering and endurance, followed by reprisal of self—a tale that holds all the information in between the lines with little given outright.

"Tell me more about yourself. How was life growing up?"

"Well, Doc, I didn't have no shiny yacht. My boat in life was that of an old jerry-rigged piece of shit. Every time I moved forward, the current would pull me back, and I did that shit for eighteen years."

"What kept pulling you off course?" I ask.

"Drugs, women, and fighting. You know, all that stupid shit us guys get into. I'd be doing good for a while and then I'd get depressed. Sometimes I'd start hearing weird shit all around me. I didn't make it any easier when I was messing around with meth either."

"So, through all that, you stayed alive and upright? Sounds like you're still fighting, but now you're fighting for all the right reasons."

"Well, brother, my mind was starting to show some serious signs of wear and tear, you know." He pauses, trying to hold back tears and keep the façade he has clung to for strength his entire life. "Now I'm fighting for sobriety, my wife, my kids, and myself."

"What else do we need, right? Family, happiness, and a clear head."

"Hell yeah!" he responds with a big smile and wide eyes no longer fixated downward in shame. "That's why I'm glad I'm here. I need to get fixed. I need you to get me back on track."

"That's my job, man, and we are going to do it together."

I decide to use this opportunity to delve further into his life and his motivating factors. "Tell me about your wife."

"Well, she is an amazing woman, but she thinks I have that multiple personality thing. My wife even made me go to therapy for it. She found a multiple personality group for me and I have been going once a week for the last month."

"Really?" I ask. "Well, which one of your personalities goes to therapy?"

He ponders the question for a split second and then breaks into laughter. "I have no fucking idea!" He continues to laugh out loud and I join him.

We continue to sit, talk, and laugh together for at least another hour, like two friends at a bar. We are as far from the label of psychiatrist and psychiatric patient as could be, even if just for a moment in time.

The next morning, I find myself exhausted in thought, running on a state of automation from the lack of sleep. The previous night's call shift was rather difficult, not allowing for respite from the chaos of residency. My legs carry me to the ward with my upper torso simply along for the ride. I'm quickly awoken as my right boot hits the door and I muster up a determined push against the heavy gate to the carnival, a carnival that is already untamed with excitement. I find myself conscious just in time to protect myself from the madness in front of and all around me. Some patients are screaming, some are pacing, and some are shadow boxing the water fountain, but all are unique, each performing an unchoreographed dance of acute mental illness. Some, however, look no different than those at a coffee shop, simply enjoying a morning conversation with an individual; unfortunately, this individual is present in form of voice or figure only heard or visible to the patient.

The mornings are always the most interesting time in the mental health hospital. Often, the last time you saw your new patient, they were distressed and suffering in this new setting of restriction, often surrounded by true madness. The "to be continued" since your last meeting may have gone well, with a dampening of the previous severity overnight. Of course, this time in waiting may have been spent simply smoldering with new symptoms awaiting to greet you when the sun rises. You concern yourself with the unknown, doing a quick chart review upon arriving. Did your patient try to end his life overnight? Did your patient try to end someone else's life overnight? Did the medications have any benefit? Any severe adverse effects? The next morning is like Christmas with all the excitement of getting a present. You could be lucky and open the wrapping to find a calm individual thanking you for all your support. It could also be less than festive; as you slowly release the ribbon, you could find yourself flat on your back with a fiery redhead on top of you trying to dismantle your nose from your face.

This morning, Abraham is one of the first patients to greet me as I push into the unit. From down the main corridor, he walks directly towards me. He gives a slight wave, which is more of a manly salute, as if to say, "Hey, let's talk." I give him an equally manly response of the head nod—a nonverbal human response mostly used in fraternities, prisons, and gangs. It's the response when an individual holds their head at its peak of motion just a millisecond longer, as if to say, "What's up?" not to be confused with the "yes" response created by a similar head motion.

"What's up, man? How are you feeling?" I casually ask.

"I feel good, Doc. Talking to you helped clear my head." His expression still remains concerned, yet I can see a glimmer of relief in his face. He appears calmer and less disturbed by the daunting task before him.

"I took those meds you gave me last night and was knocked the fuck out!"

"So, you slept well?"

"Man, I ain't slept that good in years."

"That's great. Sometimes we just need a little medication and a lot of sleep," I respond, reaffirming the benefits of the medications.

I know that this rapid of an improvement is most likely not due to pharmacological intervention and is most likely a placebo—not a placebo in the sense of a drug without an active ingredient, but a placebo driven by the mere structure and schedule of the facility, the attentive ears, and the environment of support.

It is amazing the precipitous transition a patient with mental illness can experience when the individual is absolved from outside stressors. Being placed in a controlled space where their only concerns are that of three meals, rest, and relaxation does wonders for the acute psyche. Don't get me wrong, psychiatric medications can be highly beneficial, but most take some time to provide a true physiological response. Initially however, and in the most acute phase of treatment, a placebo is organically created by a resting mind, a quiet facility, structure of wake-eat-sleep, as well as positive human interactions. This is often just enough to hold the patient steady until the medication has a chance to affect the brain's pathology, neural connections, neurotransmitter concentrations, and the receptors with which they bind.

I use this situation of artificial restoration to sanity, due to simple mental rest, as a way to reinforce the benefits of medications. This means that I convince them that their improvement is based on the medications even when I realize this may not be the entire truth. This way patients will relate their wellness to such medication and continue with medication compliance after discharge. This conformity to prescription adherence alone is a battle won very infrequently.

Abraham stays in the mental health facility for two more days, completing his 72-hour hold. I see no reason to write another hold comprised of 14 days known as a 5250. On the day of discharge, I inform him of his impending release, and he reaches out with both arms and wraps me in a hug before I can interrupt his forward progress. Most of the time I redirect such signs of affection from patients to the germ-free fist bump. Oddly, I don't do such with him as I realize it is what he needs. He needs to let me know his appreciation and I want him to know I'm not scared or repulsed by his condition. I want him to know that we are similar in many things, a sense of brotherhood for those who have experienced suffering.

I spend some time tending to other patients, adjusting medications, and partaking in my least favorite exercise of documentation. When I get a call that Abraham is ready for discharge, I head to the unit to walk him out.

"I'm ready, Doc," he states as I walk back onto the unit. He is back in the clothes he came into the emergency room wearing and no longer in the light-blue scrubs and yellow socks which designated him as a patient.

"That's awesome, brother, let's get you outta here."

"You gotta do me a favor, Doc," he states as we walk through the pair of double doors and down the long hallway to freedom.

"Sure man. What do you need?"

"I want you to come outside and meet my wife. I told her all about you and that I have a Doc with tattoos and long hair. She wants to shake your hand for all you have done for me."

"Of course. I'd love to."

We escape the final set of locked doors—yes, you counted correctly, there are three pairs of locked doors—and we find ourselves in the waiting room for family members and out the door to freedom, better known as the parking lot.

We walk up to the only car not in a spot and parked right in front next to the loading and unloading sign. His wife steps out and walks around the back of the car. We meet her at the trunk, as I assume, he will store his belongings in it during his trek. She greets me with a smile and bright-red hair not much different than the red locks worn by Abraham. A fitting bride for my new redheaded Viking comrade.

"You must be Dr. McLaughlin."

"I am. Nice to meet you." I extend my arm to shake her hand. I again find myself wrapped in her arms just as Abraham had done earlier. As she hugs me, she provides me with warm wishes of gratitude for the care I gave Abraham. I don't have the nerve to tell them how little I truly did, so instead I say, "He did all the work. He's a good man and he certainly loves his family. Take care of him." I smile and turn to shake the hand of the zombie-slaying patient I now consider a friend.

As they drive away waving, I am taken back by their gratitude with an ever-present confused look. I provided the care I should, no more, no less. I did what any mental health provider should do. I related to him, showed him respect, and simply shut my mouth and listened without judgement. It is now obvious to me where my skills lie: not in psychopharm, not in intelligence, but in relatability. I'm just your average guy who made a bunch of shitty decisions as a young man and turned his life around. I make no excuses for my past but instead let it genuinely come through, embracing it as what has molded the man I am today. I will forever be the labeled physician that rides his Harley to work and refuses to cover his tattoos. I will be unrecognizable and unrelatable to my colleagues. I will forever be the doctor that blends in all too well with the patients he treats, and I'm okay with that. In fact, I'm okay with all of it.

It's amazing the impact we can have by just being our real self and rising above the fear most physicians have of being seen as in the same categories as their patients. We as mental health providers are no better than those we treat. We were just insightful enough to follow our passion in medicine and too stubborn, or masochistic, to quit. We should treat every patient as if they are our family member or friend, and maybe then those with mental health issues will feel afforded the luxury of being related to and understood.

CHAPTER 6

Nightmares of Lucidity

TYLER

"I wish bad brain stuff was an actual guy
I could punch in the face. [. . .] Stuff's a lot harder
to fight when they're stuck in your own head."
—RoAnna Sylver

There's a brilliant flash of light, as instantaneous as the shock from an unsuspecting lightning bolt, yet with much greater overall intensity. The sound is like that of thunder, so deafening that you perceive nothing, as maybe the brain is unable to process such a concentration of force. The billowing of flames and smoke rise high above the horizon. The massive inferno, littered with ash, fashions a cloud marked as an uncultivated and ever-rising mushroom. As this pillow of death reaches the sky, continuing into the atmosphere, you experience a collection of both amazement and terror. Only later do you feel the pulse of the blast, pushing you slightly back. You witness the destruction of buildings and houses, all converted from places of family dinners and bedtime stories to silent rubble. An empty school bus, still upright and smoldering, remains parked in wait, as if to pick up children that will never arrive.

You stand alone in this wasted land of glowing destruction, the heat from the blast still radiating your skin. You look down to see the blisters arise, one by one, on your arms. Your hands are charred, and your clothing has melted, hugging every curve of your body. You are overcome by the smell of burning flesh followed by an intense feeling of sickness. Dizziness begins as your body starts to sway from its inability to gain a sense of position. You grasp your head, applying pressure in an effort to comfort the pain. You close your eyes as tightly as you can to help endure the sting, and then suddenly your eyelids retract and you find yourself back in your bedroom, both safe and free from the pain that only moments ago was gnawing at your skull. Nothing is amiss, with no radiation fallout and no sign of any destruction. You realize the trauma just suffered was only inside your mind, deprived of any indications of reality. It's then you sadly realize how complete your illness has become. It's then you realize, even without an impending end of days, your life would never again be the same; forever at odds with your own brain would be the course henceforth.

On day 3,317, I find myself stricken by a need to find a sanctuary of sorts among the outpatient psychiatric system. The lack of personnel, and limitation of resources, fashions a sense of desperation from me. The feeling of needing to heal everyone on their first visit persists throughout the day. The day is filled with just as many social issues as those of mental health origin. I do not fall into the category of people who believe that hard times, substance abuse, and homelessness create mental health disorders. I do appreciate, however, how such things can exacerbate underlying pathologies and trigger genetic predispositions.

Patient after patient steps through my door, unable to afford their medications, unable to even pick up their medications due to lack of transport. Most possess only a limited ability to care for themselves. Most are consumed simply by discovering an opportunity for a hot meal and the comfort of a roof over their head. I try to find the importance of mental wellness amid the suffering of everyday life.

Many of my patients who are forced to rely on county outpatient clinics wear their suffering in their expression. A story in itself is carved into the worn frowns and lines of their faces. When tattered clothing is upon their body and there is an overall display of hunger and distress, I look away from solving psychiatric issues. I find myself engaged in more social work than my initial intended medical intervention. I try to focus my attention on the positive, finding myself a fool, determined to make a one-man stand against the limited nationwide mental health care system one patient at a time.

My current patient will be my last patient of the day, and unfortunately, the eye-opening experience is enough to make up for an entire week of disappointment. This is a patient who would re-fuel my belief in the human condition jailed in a disorder. He is a person with an organ hell-bent on complicating his mere existence and perception with all that is present. He gives me what I crave to see yet am saddened to watch: suffering housed in the brain. His is a condition with organic etiologies and not those exacerbated by tumultuous life experiences.

Tyler is a well-spoken young man of only 20 years of age when he is presented to my outpatient clinic. Tyler is one of the most interesting individuals I will ever meet. Upon first arriving at my office, he appears greatly disheveled and unkempt. He was transported from a group home "for the psychiatrically ill" by a camp counselor and simply dropped off like a five-year-old child being escorted to his classroom by staff. His clothing is an eclectic mess of colors, as if he had hurriedly dressed in the dark. Neither of his shoes are properly tied, and I have to restrain the urge to kneel down and simply tie them for him. Appearing unshaved for weeks, his beard is patchy and ungroomed. His posture is slightly hunched over, with a slow and purposeful gait appearing careful not to engage in sudden movements. He displays rigidity in the turning of his head from one side to another. Not quite torticollis, but more of what one would witness in someone with a neck brace on.

He greats me in a calm and almost relaxing voice. His speech is somewhat impaired by a mild case of voice cracking, and I assume he is just nervous. I invite him to have a seat across from me on the other side of the lightly tanned, shabby, particle board desk. I make the normal introductions explaining who I am, my role, and of course a statement regarding confidentiality. I have to disclose to patients that whatever they tell me will remain between the two of us. I basically can serve as a priest during your confession; however, this priest cannot absolve you from your sins, only medicate you. You can literally confess to a previous murder and I can't utter a word.

The doctor-patient privilege, especially in the field of psychiatry, is imperative and solid in its standards. Only in circumstances of ongoing child or elder abuse, as well as those circumstances which present as an imminent threat to either the patient or the public, can such lines of privilege be crossed. These cases of abuse and imminent threats encompass either a threat to harm self or others, and all fall outside of doctor-patient privilege, as I am required to report such cases. In some circumstances, a patient may admit to a bank robbery he committed ten years prior and where he buried the loot, and this will undoubtedly stay without a voice of expression to anyone other than myself. However, if someone tells me of their impending plan to execute another, I am forced to report it to authorities. I am also mandated to make every attempt to notify and warn the intended victim. This is considered a duty to warn also known as the Tarasoff duty. This was not always the case and it took an unfortunate, and unnecessary, loss of life before this ruling came aboard.

Tyler makes an effort to respond to my initial statements with fringes of active listening, often nodding his head to statements he understands. His speech begins to slowly describe a multitude of somatic complaints involving generalized pain and sedation. It is obvious he is unclear as to my role and most likely has mistaken me for his primary care provider. I step back to reaffirm the reason for our meeting and how I hope our therapeutic relationship will flourish.

Tyler seems to understand, and I quickly become the ear to all his inner workings and frustrations. This is rare, to have someone engrain their trust in you so quickly, but I think the answers to his questions involving perception of reality have been wearing on him for quite some time. He does not want to waste any more of his future hidden behind the unknown and is searching for a friend to help him find his way.

Tyler begins to divulge his most personal, and often unique, symptoms of mental distress, and each seems more devastating than the last. I wonder how he even survived this long with the insurmountable detachment from reality that he has been coping with.

One such symptom is explicitly distressing and something entirely foreign to my experience and knowledge. He explains that his mind has created an unwillingness for contact, bordering on a physical inability towards contact. This is not for fear of germs, as is all too common in our current age of antibiotics and hand sanitizers, but for something much more ominous. Whether it be for objects or to even shake hands, he has the perception that his distinctive being could, and often did, become fused with that of another person or object. He tells me about often finding himself attached to objects while feeling an inability to tear himself away.

Tyler explains, "My hand will touch a table or a doorknob and it's almost as if the molecular structure of my cells bond with the molecular structure of the object. It's like the cells of my hand fit perfectly into the microscopic grooves of the object. It's like a gecko's foot. Sometimes I can't unpair the junction of my hand for minutes."

The feeling that upon touching an object, a person's molecular structure would become embedded within the surface of the object, not allowing for release, is considered a tactile hallucination. Tales of being stuck to a table for several minutes due to this phenomenon, while interesting to the listener, has caused Tyler severe anxiety, and must have been nothing short of terrifying. This knowledge now explains the awkward hand and arm position with which he currently presents himself. Both of his arms are held close to the body. What I initially felt was potentially a display of upper extremity rigidity may in fact be purposeful to limit his incidental contact. His paranoia guides his arms to the flexed position, with hands out in front, palms up and facing his own body. It is as if he just scrubbed in for surgery and is attempting to keep the sterile field of his hands intact as he awaits gowning and gloves.

As we continue to discuss, we go deeper into the emotional price his disorder has cost. As he becomes more comfortable with me, I feel the invitation to delve further. I want to know not only how his brain has affected his function, but also how his reality has suffered from such impairment. His mind has interpreted a reality of disorganization and fragmentation; however, his insight into his illness is intact. This is a unique setting, seeing both the trees and the forest. This duality primes the individual to an increased rate of comorbid depressive disorder.

In my experience, depression is often present as a product of intelligent insight into psychiatric illness and as a condition most prevalent in those persons with a highly functional, premorbid condition. In those individuals with above-average intellect and many premorbid aspirations and dreams, the impact of schizophrenia is most severe to the delicate component of self. The illness slowly creeps in, known as the prodrome phase, first disturbing their relationships, motivations, grades, and sleep patterns. The sufferers tell themselves that this is just a normal life phase or even possibly a bacterial or viral illness that will remain short-lived. Hope for quick resolution begins to dissolve as the individual begins to experience delusions of paranoia as well as hallucinations, auditory or visual, and even the rarer perceptual disturbance of tactile hallucinations, as seen in Tyler's case. Further into the illness, with self-realization of mounting cognitive functional impairments, the maintained insight into the illness, its chronicity, and the impact on normalcy impart a decisive blow to the dreams and aspirations once held.

I allow him time to just process, out loud, some of his experiences, which he executes in a calm and educated voice yet with extreme intensity. It's as if I'm listening to someone reading a fictional novel, but in this instance, the characters and the mystifying occurrences they face are all real inside Tyler's mind.

I give guidance regarding structure to our encounter. "I want you to tell me some of the experiences that you have been facing. Let's start with the most frightening and we will move from there to those events that are not as bad."

Tyler begins to dictate his experiences, and I am all ears. Looking back, I feel guilty for having such excitement in hearing detailed accounts of his brain's betrayal. "When it's bad, it's like jumping into a fire. Like watching a nuclear explosion with everything crumbling. I can feel the energy pulse through my body. For that moment, my limbs actually feel warm, as if I can feel the heat from the blast. I can smell the smoldering structures. I see a vivid scene of destruction. I have to assure myself it's not the apocalypse and that it's just in my head. When it's not that bad, it's like a computer. It's hard to describe, but I guess the best way is to say it resembles a computer screen. The display is three-dimensional, and each shape represents a file. The shapes glow on a background of a computer screen." As he says this, his arms raise, and his finger reaches out to touch something in his field of view that only he can see.

"Can you click on these glowing images?" I ask.

"Yes. Like right now, I just touched one. When I touch one, it lights up brighter and opens another folder. I know in reality it's not in front of me. I know it's in my mind, but the experience feels very real to me. There is a connector that comes from the display. It's like a bunch of wires. They are running beneath me almost like a power cord." His gaze and attention are mirrored by his arm movements as he follows this power cord from his field of view to its course next to him, continuing to document its placement as it runs behind him and through the wall of my office. "The lines and cords are running systematically all over like you're looking into a computer switchboard. It's really strange. Sometimes I see shapes I have never seen before and sometimes I hear music, in my mind, that I have never heard before. It just so strange, but interesting at the same time."

Impressed by his command of language and his attention to details, my curiosity takes over and I ask for further interpretation. "Do you ever feel like the things you see are more than just manifestations of your mind? Do you ever feel like you're trapped in something outside of normal human consciousness, or something outside of the typical human perspective?"

"Honestly, I have considered the possibility, however remote, that I'm experiencing something real, but the greater part of me knows it's not."

"Can you tell me about when these experiences began?" I ask.

"It was gradual. I can almost trace the origin to seven or eight years ago. I had this thing I called 'material senses.' I would have these concepts. These concepts would turn into concrete pictures in my mind. I would see these images overlaid in my visual field. The philosophical questions regarding the universe, and life in general, were eating me alive. Things got really bad about a year ago and led to severe anxiety."

"So, when you can recall the origins of these material senses, can you remember if anything pivotal was going on? Any particular stressor or traumatic experience coinciding with such origination?"

"Well, five years ago, my mom died of brain cancer. I was living in Seattle at the time. I couldn't really work after she died, I assume from grief or depression. Subsequently, I got into some financial trouble, so I had to move down here where more family is located."

"I am so very sorry to hear about the loss of your mother. That must have been very difficult on you."

"It was hard, and it came on rather sudden. Maybe the sudden nature of the cancer was part of the reason it was so difficult."

"What about before that? Before your mother died." I continue to search for reason. I remain motivated, or better yet, forced to find meaning behind the cause of suffering in such an intelligent and innocent soul.

"The only thing I can think of is that I was obsessing. I mean, I still do that today, but not with the same magnitude. I would sit in my room all day, just thinking about intellectual topics. It would generate stress. Going back to middle school and high school, it was never as bad back then. I can't really tell you how far it goes back, but in hindsight, I feel like it was always there."

We continue to chat for the better part of two hours. As our time nears its completion, we discuss interventions and develop a plan to add mental stability to his menu of entrees. Also, I give him the list of testing that I do with anyone suffering from new-onset psychosis, or in a patient with chronic psychotic symptoms who has never been under the care of a psychiatrist.

So, what does a psychiatrist order when you arrive at his or her office with psychotic features? This list is sizeable, but the most important items are a CT scan of the brain as a preliminary diagnostic tool. This helps to rule out intracranial processes such as tumor, infarction, hemorrhage, or other viral and parasitic processes. An electrocardiogram (ECG or EKG) is ordered to check the function, and the conduction, of the heart. Many of our antipsychotics can create a prolonging of the QT interval, basically meaning that these drugs can kill you if you have an underlying cardiac conduction anomaly. Next are the basic labs including electrolyte, metabolic, and lipid profiles. Measurement of body weight and vital signs (heart rate, blood pressure, temperature) is also recommended. Other laboratory tests to be considered are a CBC (complete blood count), fasting glucose levels, as well as tests of liver, renal, and thyroid function. An RPR (syphilis test), HIV test, as well as a good 'ol urine drug screen is essential. For women of childbearing age, a pregnancy test must also be considered.

In patients for whom the clinical picture is unclear, or in cases of abnormal findings from these routine examinations, more detailed studies (e.g., screening for heavy metal toxicity, electroencephalogram, or MRI scan) may be indicated. In cases of psychosis where schizophrenia is also suspected, the conduction of speedy testing, when possible, is of the utmost importance. The goal is to determine etiology and initiate treatment for symptoms of schizophrenia in its initial episode as soon as possible.

When a patient presents with a first-episode psychosis, regardless of age, close observation, history of illness through collateral information, and documentation of the signs and symptoms over time are important. First episodes of psychosis can be polymorphic and evolve into a variety of specific disorders (e.g., schizophreniform disorder, bipolar disorder, schizoaffective disorder).

Also important to consider, in any potential psychotic disorder, is the risk of suicide. It remains imperative to assess for suicide risk at all stages of the illness and to perform an initial suicide risk assessment and regular evaluation of suicide risk as part of each patient's psychiatric assessment. We screen for a multitude of symptoms and identification of risk factors for potential suicidality, and still, despite our best efforts, it remains impossible to predict whether an individual patient will attempt suicide, and all we can do is adjust our calculated perception of risk for such.

I was lucky enough to follow Tyler's case for the next 12 months, becoming what I like to believe an instrumental part in his recovery and constancy. Ever so slowly his symptoms lessened. The impairment on his proper function was so decreased in severity that we actually discussed plans for him to get his own place. Functioning as an individual, he would learn to cope as any young man, or young woman, leaving the security of their parent's home. I hoped that instead of residing in a home as a group and being attached with a label, he could return to his old life and just be Tyler. I hoped his greatest concern would be that of finding love and which college degree to work towards instead of battling persistent symptoms of a chronically debilitating illness. Simply being a young man with opportunities abounding and a bright future is all I wished for him. I said a proud goodbye to my newfound friend as residency calls for constant change with limited continuity of care. Once your year of outpatient psychiatry is over, you are forced to move to new rotations to fill required experiences. The patients you grow to care about become someone else's problem and you are just a distant memory.

I never did see him again, and I hope his life is flourishing from inside his mind. I hope he will one day meet a girl and go back to college. I hope that his dreams and goals are achieved and that he finds happiness and fulfillment in all he deserves. As I recount this story on parchment, I hope the words in this chapter are nothing more than a distant memory for Tyler, memories that will soon be placed aside for more fruitful and beautiful exposures of human growth and happiness.

CHAPTER 7

What's Buggin' You?

NANCY

"There's nothing worse than being betrayed by your confidant, your companion, your best friend, yourself."

The belief that a person is infected with parasites of the skin, invisible to the naked eye, is no less probable than the white orb found in the Christmas photo your grandma swears is your late uncle Bernie, as she explains, "Of course it's him. Bernie just loved the holidays." Yet, with that being said, low probability does not rule out possibility. Therefore, as a physician, all is possible until it's ruled out.

When approached scientifically, the information provided to the patient by the doctor has to be processed and accepted prior to treatment. Treatments, regardless of their proven efficacy, are only as good as the mind believes it to be. Just as the brain influences the mind, the mind can also pave roads for the brain. These pathways are for the brain to follow in hopes of guiding function to meet expectations. The patient's mind has to make the decision to find validity in the presence of a strong emotion, either for the physician's diagnosis or to reject the diagnosis and seek their own path to truth. Seeing something through the goggles of wanting to believe can often make the trivial seem significant.

Delusions are a facet of psychosis that can be that of a singular, yet particular, false belief. Some individuals can remain delusional their entire life and can function completely normal in society. Some believe they have the ability to read tea leaves while others believe the Earth is only 5000 years young. Both of these individuals will most likely never see the inside of a mental health hospital and may function as stellar members of the community. Some may even step into the role of teacher or minister, charged with rejecting evolution and spreading their delusions to the masses. Others, however, can have delusions that are much more devastating to the sufferer. Some may have misconceptions of infestations, via parasites or bugs, and completely disintegrate into nothing but a faint shell of their former self. A delusion is fixed into the psyche and even a singular delusion can become chronic, fashioning a web that entangles a person's entire life, encompassing and slowly smothering all that they hold dear.

It's a horrible thing to watch a human's reality crash before them. The once stable and carefree wife and mother now shattered into shards of what they believe to be truth, losing not only their sanity, but their loved ones, their friends and support systems, their jobs, and their individuality. Their place in society becomes that of the unwanted crazies, and with it they must force their delusions to be hidden, burying their beliefs along with their former life. Often those delusions do not lie dead and resurface to construct a whole new person fixated only on his or her plight, defined only by their struggle and their need to have others believe so that they may once again take their rightful place in the tribe.

I was able to witness all of the above struggles manifested into one poor soul when Nancy, a forty-something mother, wife, and substitute teacher for grades K through 6, walked into the local emergency room for treatment.

It was day 3365, and I happened to be the acting resident psychiatrist in that emergency department.

The story began as I opened my ice-cold energy drink. I had found a place of momentary rest as I peacefully perched on a stool hidden in the corner of the emergency department. As I'm about to take my first refreshing drink of caffeine and chemicals, which I have grown quite fond of, I am painfully interrupted. It is as though someone heard the crisp inaugural opening of the can and decided an intervention into my moment of Zen was required. As I look up, my lips pursed and still affixed to the can, I see both the emergency department resident and his attending staring at me from a rather uncomfortable distance. They obviously do not adhere to the widely practiced crotch-to-face distance rule of at least 48 inches. At any given time, I prefer my face to be at least four feet from the nearest crotch in the room.

"We got one we would like you to consult on," the resident says speedily as he can notice my slight displeasure in the interruption.

"Okay, what do we have?" I slowly stand up as to not have my head strike the attending's invading pelvic area on my way up. Using my right leg, I politely push my stool back with a single shove. I let the wind of the attending's lungs push me rearward so that I can keep my mind focused on the case presentation and not on discerning what flavor of gum is being willfully expressed in the direction of my face. They both seem exhausted with just the short time spent with the patient, and they appear more than happy to request a psych consult.

"We have no idea what the hell is going on with her. She is cleared from a medical standpoint, but maybe you guys can take her," suggests the attending as he remains stoic in his long, and rather stiff, pressed white coat.

When another non-psychiatric physician says, "Maybe you guys can take them," that's code for, "We have no idea what is wrong with the patient, so it must be psych-related. Can you please get them the fuck away from me because they are doing a bang-up job of creeping me out? On second thought, please go hide them in the mental health hospital!"

I gather myself and head in the direction of the room, not staying long enough during the case presentation to even get the room, as I figured, "Well, I have her name, so I'll just wing it."

I start glancing into each room through the glass sliding doors. I'm not sure what good I am doing just peering into a room for half a second, hoping to determine if they are a psychiatric patient by sight alone.

Just then I hear a female voice say, "Doctor."

I look in the direction of the voice and see an ER nurse, leaning over her computer, smiling and pointing to the glass cage two down from where I'm standing. I give her a smile in acknowledgement of her assistance and softly knock on the outside of the enclosure.

"Come in," a woman's voice shouts out.

I notice the shades have been partly drawn closed by the medical staff, so I enter with caution, hoping all orifices are covered with some sort of clothing. I first open the heavy and rather bulky glass sliding door and ever so carefully pull to the side the tan, banana-patterned curtain, realizing that hearing the words, "Come in," does not always coincide with appropriate clothing. I walk in and am initially glad to see an individual fully clothed and not in her birthday suit looking to coerce the next doctor that comes in. There will be no fulfillment of some Fifty-Shades-of-Grey type of fantasy today, nor a re-enactment of the promiscuity seen on Grey's Anatomy.

I walk in to find a rather normal-appearing woman in her mid-forties, standing anxiously among her spread of organized chaos. She has made quick work of the small exam room and turned it into a museum of subjective horrors. Before I have the chance to describe my role or provide credentials, she begins to state her case.

"I've lost everything because of this, because of these bugs. I need you to look at these." She is crying out as if something is on fire and I need to put it out.

Nancy presents a wide array of pictures to me. The pictures number in the hundreds and she did her best to spread them over the exam table. One by one, they are laid out in rows of obvious proof. She stands next to the scene like a representative at a trade show, displaying her new products. I notice many of the pictures are Polaroid, and I can't help but wonder where in the hell she dug up such an old piece of equipment.

I begin to glance at them one by one, each out-of-focus picture obviously taken at very close range to the skin. Such a photo will often cause a blur in focus with the attempted magnification of the most innocuous material. The blurring of a definitive outline leaves the identity of such an impression wide open to interpretation. For those looking for bugs, these pictures provide a target-rich environment: a canvas of skin with a plethora of distorted images all subjectively presented as more ominous than the last. Looking at her pictures reminds me of looking up at the clouds with my young son, both of us detailing to each other our interpretations of the wondrous mixture of gas, liquids, and solids floating above us.

In addition to the photographic proof supplied, she also provides many forms of physical specimens for which she apparently wants me to examine. Each specimen is housed in plastic bags, some Ziploc and some simply in cheap, fold-over sandwich bags, hastily closed at the top with a knot. Also present are samples of fibrous strands, folded into pieces of packing tape. She has designated these pieces of physical evidence to the counter of the cabinet housing the sink. The items captured on adhesive tape, as one would do when clearing lint from an item of clothing, are no more enlightening than the previous specimens. These too, unfortunately, appear to contain nothing more than purposeful placement of misunderstood lint and hair samples. I do my best to not show my hand and further decompensate her trust in medical professionals. I do all the necessary moans, gasps, and head nodding indicative of a man deeply intent on discovering a clue—a clue that she yearns for me to notice and accept. I feel her eyes fixated on my facial expressions, trying to gather insight into my inner debate. The only way I can make it through the hundreds of specimens and not display my position of psychiatric illness over infestation is to momentarily accept what I see through her own eyes. Only through the mimicking of belief can I act my way through these moments of discomfort.

For thousands of years, the notion of a village gave a sense of safety. When suffering from delusions, we search for such safety via validation from the experiences of others. We are wired to search for information, be it newspaper articles or online sites, that coincides with our own beliefs. Through mirroring, we only further delve into a sense of justification, a justification often found in groups of individuals with a common belief or ideology. No one wants to be the only person who believes in a conspiracy. We are tormented to extend our knowledge to others, even when we, ourselves, question its validity. All this to ease the burden and garner confirmation in our personal convictions.

On further inspection of the physical specimens provided, I find what I believe to be a mixture of clothing lint, pieces of dry skin, and other simple household debris. I can make no definitive recognition of any foreign biological material, and trust me, I wanted to find some. It would be so much more interesting to discover some rare infestation burrowing itself into human skin rather than the admission that her suffering is that of the brain and nothing that we can see, measure, or extract. How I wish it was a case of parasites or bugs or any obvious biological infiltration. An infiltration by a known genus with some sort of well-known treatment would indemnify my patient back to her stable self and do so in rapid measure. In fact, that's one reason we, as psychiatrists, look for pathological causes of symptoms mimicking mental illness. The pathological causes are usually much more straightforward and simpler to treat.

Treating mental illness is difficult both in its identification and its constructs of being multifaceted in origination. It is more of an art, using out-of-the-box thinking to treat complex brain derangements with psychopharmacology.

To make matters worse, this psychopharmacology toolbox, utilized to treat, is often done so with the knowledge of our limitations on how each medication actually works. To further complicate the process, we are often forced to step outside the safety of FDA approval and use off-label strategies to attack obscure and refractory cases.

In the short time that we spent together, I can only speculate on the duration and course of such a condition. Maybe it was the delusions that led to her debility, or maybe the delusions were easier to accept than the truth of having a mental disorder. Maybe her downfall wasn't only a product of mental illness but also due to a brittle sense of self, unable or unwilling to accept a diagnosis so ingrained with attached stigma. Maybe there was even something of much greater depth at work here.

I take a quick hiatus to find the patient's family and gather some collateral. Her husband, whom she is legally separated from, as well as her teenage son, greet me as I enter the waiting room. We find a safe place to talk. I am provided with a barrage of trauma faced by Nancy that would certainly drive any of us insane. Her reported past begins to shed possible light into the patient's current suffering.

Upon exploration into the time of onset, I learn that in the months before her "break from reality," she had a small stent of time, approximately six months, when she was treated with antipsychotics for new-onset auditory hallucinations. These auditory hallucinations were of rapid onset and coincided with severe depression. Driving her pain were perceptual disturbances of auditory content of two men talking about all the ways they tortured and raped her 19-year-old daughter. According to family, shortly before Nancy began to suffer from changes in mental state, her daughter, freshly off to college, had been kidnapped, raped, and tortured. Her daughter, newly acquainted to the evil that is man, decided her life was worth nothing if she didn't have supreme say of who was allowed to touch her. Her daughter decided to abandon the labor of motion within a life void of comfort.

The undiluted heartbreak that Nancy felt when she later found her daughter hanging in the garage must have been unbearable, to say the least. The only indication of her daughter's suicide was the residual of a fallen chair and the high-pitch squeaks from the wooden crossbeams. A noise of unfortunate consequence originated by the shifting of human weight. Death's ominous, last song played by a lifeless composer swaying back and forth. An artist still tethered to Earth, yet ultimately free from all but gravity.

The note, left neatly folded and upright on her bed upstairs, added little to console Nancy's pain. Although the letter stated at one point, "Please don't blame yourself; this is my choice," she would continue to do just that, then and in every moment of every day since then. The void that marked that juncture in time would be one without fathom and endless in its depth. I can only imagine this darkness as being more than a time without light but instead comprising a complete absence of faith.

"She never became quite whole again," her husband adds. "She just couldn't stop blaming herself for what happened."

I walk back into the exam room feeling so sorry for Nancy that I can barely look her in the eye for fear of breaking down in front of her. It's now slightly clearer that her current presentation may be an indication of the guilt she has placed upon herself to endure. Maybe the infestation on her body was a mere reflection of the internal lack of worth she felt. A mirrored termination of self-significance. A life of condemnation doomed to be that as flesh buried below the ground; bound to be nothing more than food for the maggots.

"I'm not crazy. These things in my skin and on my body are real. Just look at the pictures. They're all over me. I'm being tormented night and day. No one believes me." She scratches methodically and unknowingly at the fragile and reddened skin of her forearms.

I push the lump down in my throat. I hold back the watery constructs gathering in my eyes and look away until I have garnered my composure. I have a bad habit of trying to relate to individuals in order to understand and help them. I try to envision what they see, feel, or hear. With that same perspective, I now have an image ingrained in my mind as I attempt to rejoin the conversation. I see myself standing in her place, in the garage, exactly where her feet stopped in horror, looking upon a young innocent girl now lifeless in form.

I gather myself and attempt to distract my own mind by asking to see her arms. Inspection of Nancy's skin does display multiple rashes and sores in different stages of healing and injury. These rashes, however, appear without the tell-tale sign of infections by bugs. There is also no evidence of psoriasis or some autoimmune disease. Some areas appear to be freshly injured with no underlying rash that itches but instead a delusional itch that rashes. The sensations she describes, leading to extensive pruritis (itching), is that of bugs crawling, also known as formication, on and under the skin. Individuals tormented by such a delusion often feel as though insects are crawling on the body or under the skin.

Now, before I can dissolve the barriers her illness has formatted, I must first assume a physiological etiology for such severe pruritis. With that being said, initial medical assessments would include a blood test with complete blood counts to rule out iron deficiency, which can lead to itching, as well as tests of thyroid, liver, and kidney function to exclude such conditions as hyperthyroidism, which may also cause itching.

In cases similar to Nancy's, patients are driven to digging out, collecting, and photo logging the fibers, threads, or stringy material they happen to find in, and on, the skin. These materials are presumed to be insects, worms, or bugs, depending on their size and shape. This scourge is surmised to have origin that is organic, via the person who desperately wishes for such. The desire for such is so great that the patient is fixed in belief despite evidence to the contrary. Unfortunately, these collections of unknowns are more likely to be that of lint, threads from clothing or other fibrous, non-biological material. These materials are violently scratched and embedded into the underlying layers of skin and into previous dermal injuries. When self-extracting such items, patients fail to realize the itching they previously engaged in likely embedded material into the already broken skin.

The intense itching and open sores associated with this disorder can substantially interfere with a person's quality of life. If severe, such a delusion can take management of all of the brain's non-automated functions, abducting the sufferer's previous life, while shattering it into small pieces and flushing them down the proverbial toilet of hope.

Most will never see a case such as delusional parasitosis, and by the end of my residency, I had unfortunately seen it twice. Delusional parasitosis, also known as Ekbom syndrome or Morgellons disease, is manifested in the patient's firm belief that he or she is suffering from an infestation with some sort of insect or parasite.

Returning from my own mind, I begin to steer the conversation towards questions involving mental illness. Looking into her eyes, not as a doctor to a patient but as a human to a human, I say, "I can see that you're suffering, and my only goal is to try to help you. I'm not here to judge, or even to diagnose your condition. My sole purpose is to understand your suffering so I can attempt to lift some of the burden."

She pauses and then quickly looks me directly in the eye. "People think I'm crazy and no one believes me. Do you believe me?"

I think to myself about a proper response to such a loaded question. Do I potentially harm the patient's delicate sense of self, further widening the divide from the help she so requires, or do I further cement her delusional convictions?

"Well, I do believe you are suffering," I say slowly, choosing every syllable correctly yet knowing this answer often sparks rage in most patients. I proceed further inward. "I'm going to ask you a question and I want you to take no offense from it. Think of my question as just being a simple question from a guy attempting to do his due diligence, while gathering a history of what you're dealing with." I pause for dramatic effect and to find the courage to speak such sacrilege in obvious desecration of her self-indoctrinated observations. Sometimes being the voice of reason can be misinterpreted as being critical of other beliefs; therefore, I tread lightly.

"Do you feel that, within all your suffering, there is any chance that the bugs may not be real?" I ask her, holding my breath in favor of a cautious exhale. "I mean, you have already gone through so much that it makes me wonder if this could all be something else at its core."

It's at this moment that our eyes meet in an understanding. Her fear to admit and commit to a logical excuse would only place the loss of her daughter back to the forefront. She begins to sob, and then I realize that, for her, maybe she felt calmer being a patient then being a mourning mother.

I know all too well that any explorations of inner workings can create emotional reactivity taking the patient from their comfort zone and back into the fire. Throughout my thoughts, she continues to cry, and within her moment of tearfulness, she abruptly stops and asks, "What are you going to do? Are you going to put me on some crazy-person meds? Meds that are going to make me drool and turn me into a zombie?"

I ponder the reason why people refer to psychiatric medications as drool-inducing zombie capsules. That's such bullshit. Sure, with heavy doses I can make you lie in bed, covering your light-blue bib with saliva. Sure, I can make you so sedated that the words you try to utter sound like the grunts and moans of a drunken sailor after celebrating a return to port. Yet, those doses are saved for only the very worst psychiatric cases, typically found in psychiatric state hospitals. In those cases, patients display severe and potentially deadly, psychosis-induced aggression. They are the patients who wish to chew your face off and wear it as a mask. I hardly think turning Nancy into a sack of drooling meat with a heartbeat on a gurney is going to fix her problems.

Rather than give her the ramblings of a mad psychiatrist, I look to her and simply say, "I would never give you medications that would do that to you. I am simply here to help you clear your thoughts and overcome what you're suffering from."

It's at this time that I explain to her and guide her through the details of multiple medications that we call antipsychotics. The name antipsychotic has got to be one of the worst drug class identifiers. To explain to someone who may be currently irrational that they require such a class of drugs will itself strike a deep sense of apprehension and fear. Such a medication designation can invoke a frightful subjective burden that life is somehow destined to be drowned in the deep end of mental illness.

In certain populations, to lessen the blow, I refer to these medications as neuroleptics and discard the stigma-provoking title of antipsychotic. People don't appreciate being associated with any word related to psychosis, nor being referred to as psychotic.

"I have tried those before, and I didn't like them."

I search for a way to convince Nancy as to the effectiveness of such medications in her current state, adding that the antipsychotic will only be a "peppering," an adjunct treatment modifier only furthering the effectiveness of our primary medication choice. The real life-changing medication will be that of the antidepressant such as seen in patients suffering from major depressive disorder with psychotic features. Yes, Nancy has a secondary delusional disorder; however, the inciting factor leading to her spiral from reality was birthed in the absolute sorrow of depression.

Now, there are a couple of small studies that were done a few years back that indicate some neuroleptics may have antiparasitic benefits. So, I use this angle and attempt to add a new scope of perspective with this information. I present these facts to her, not as a form of trickery, but as a form of option. With this theoretical potential for intervention into her fixed belief, I have provided her fragile sense of self the option of believing the use of antipsychotics is exclusively for her parasitic skin infection, in the hope this will create a state of lessened concern for the stigma accompanying such medication use.

Antipsychotic medications are commonly used to treat your basic psychosis-related disturbances including generalized disorganization that is represented by symptoms of hallucinations and non-linear thought process; however, in the current state of medicine, they are also used for mood stabilization in bipolar disorder, aggression, violence refractory to other interventions, and even insomnia. There are also times when antipsychotics will be prescribed off-label for seemingly less intuitive issues such as hiccups and headaches and in even more rare instances for their properties of reduced growth in parasitic infestations and for their anti-pruritic properties.

Most practitioners and scientists have ignored the potential underlying causes responsible for formication and beliefs of infestation. It is easier to declare mental illness the exclusive etiologic cause, thus blaming the patient when confronted with perplexing and unexplained symptoms. However, it is irresponsible to label a patient delusional without a complete medical assessment and only then with an appropriate psychiatric evaluation. If mental illness is presumed to be present, a physician should bear in mind that an underlying infectious process can certainly cause a pathological response which itself may result in symptoms indicative of, or mimicking, a mental illness. It is the possibility of underlying infectious process that is the crux in the equation. Do you feel an infectious process is a possibility or do your feel the brain has once again trumped the mind in this hand of delusional poker?

When diagnosing mental illness, it is imperative to first determine if there is an underlying medical cause of the psychiatric symptoms—and not in just some patients, but in every patient. Therefore, calling for a psychiatric evaluation after five minutes with a patient is simply ridiculous. Rather than just going along with the flow of the river of complacency and laziness, I instead often decide to cut down a tree and dam that river up. Prior to discharge, I will make sure Nancy receives full blood workup, laboratory and microscopy of skin biopsies, as well as the provided unknown fibrous evidence. This will be in addition to a urine drug screen, autoimmune titers, and head imaging—quite the expensive workup, all thanks to the psychiatric resident.

Delusional parasitosis and its symptoms are nothing new, and it has been described in the medical literature for over 75 years. The false belief of parasitic infestation stands in contrast to actual cases of parasitosis, such as scabies, which has a fairly consistent presentation of small sores in the webbing between the fingers, but which may also appear in any area of skin where these little mites burrow into your flesh causing severe itching and pain.

People suffering from delusional parasitosis are likely to first seek help not from psychiatrist, but from dermatologists. Such a condition is not well known to all medical providers, and therefore there may be circumstances where the illness is incorrectly diagnosed clinically by the patient's primary care provider. This primary care provider will often refer to dermatology as the obvious next step in course of care. When said dermatological assessment arrives at a subsequent psychiatric referral the patient will often seek out a new primary care provider to validate his or her claims of infestation and the cycle continues. It's safe to say that a psychiatrist will never meet a person with delusional parasitosis who hasn't first worn out all local dermatologists and primary care physicians.

Nancy's case had become so severe that she was basically participating in self-mutilation. As she rolls up the sleeves of her shirt for me, large areas of her flesh are reddened from the persistent scratching and picking. Some of her skin is blackened and scarred from attempts to exorcise the parasitic demons with a butter knife she would hold over an open stovetop flame. The most worrisome areas are that of her abdomen. Just a slight lifting of her shirt to display the area around the umbilicus (a.k.a. the bellybutton) reveals fresh superficial lacerations and others that are much deeper. Part of the skin covering her stomach has actually been cut away, with large deeps scars and scabs present due to her own inexperienced surgical handiwork. She details further rituals, which are less invasive but just as dangerous and include bathing with a large percentage of her bathwater comprised of bleach and pouring isopropyl alcohol over her body to kill the bacteria that she feels were produced by the creatures infesting her.

At this point, my ideas of discharge to outpatient psychiatry dissolve and I begin to feel a 5150 is needed to stabilize her and give her a place where we can monitor her for safety. Individuals with delusional disorders do not typically require inpatient psychiatric hospitalization; however, the severity of her self-mutilation gives me a clear sense that she is a current danger to self. In her attempts to rid herself of her microscopic captures, she has fortunately given me cause to admit her. This may be the best chance for her to gain hold of reality and bid herself adieu to the psychosis that has plagued and literally scarred her.

Nancy's condition is not one of complete rarity, as such presentations have worried the medical community for years. In fact, over the last 20 years, a multitude of studies and financial grants have set out to explore all possible biological options prior to discarding such interpretations as falsehoods. A study conducted of 108 patients at the Mayo Clinic was published in the Archives of Dermatology on May 16, 2011. The study was unable to find evidence of skin infestation despite doing skin biopsies and examining specimens provided by over 100 self-reported patient infestations.

Even the Center for Disease Control set out to investigate such occurrences. The report was labeled *The CDC Investigation of Morgellons*. This interest by the CDC was only after a mailing campaign coordinated by the Morgellons Research Foundation in which self-described sufferers were able to log into the affiliated website and send what amounted to thousands of form letters to members of Congress. The CDC task force first met in June 2006. The task force consisted of 12 people, including two pathologists, a toxicologist, an ethicist, a mental health expert, and specialists in the fields of infectious, parasitic, environmental, and chronic diseases.

In June 2007, the CDC opened a website, and by November of 2007 they had announced the beginning of an active investigation process, stating, "The primary goals of the investigation are to better describe the clinical and epidemiologic features of this condition and to generate hypotheses about possible risk factors." Kaiser Permanente in Northern California was chosen to assist with the investigation. Investigators planned to report on the geographic distribution of the illness and estimate rates of illness in affected communities. The investigation involved skin biopsies from affected patients and characterization of foreign material such as fibers or threads obtained from patients to determine their potential source.

In January 2008, it was reported that the CDC was enlisting the aid of the U.S. Armed Forces Institute of Pathology and the American Academy of Dermatology to "conduct immediate and rigorous research."

On January 25, 2012, the CDC released the results of the study they conducted on unexplained dermopathy (a.k.a. Morgellons disease). Findings of the study described no infectious or environmental links. The study consisted of skin biopsies, blood tests, and interviews and yielded no evidence of infection or infestation. Analysis of the threads provided by participants was proven to consist of cotton and other materials likely to be found in clothing.

Various Morgellons groups responded to the results of the studies by saying it confirmed their expectations that the government-run studies were trying to cover up larger issues, suggesting a conspiracy of sorts. A large website related to Morgellons disease sufferers, which hosts theories on the causes of Morgellons, even went as far as to suggest symptoms possibly being related to alien implants.

I am not one to judge, as I personally have not conducted any in-depth physical research. I can only diagnose what I see, in the context of what I do not see. I keep an open mind to all possibilities, but for now, regarding Nancy, all the data, or lack thereof, points to a diagnosis that could simply be labeled as suffering. I complete the 5150 paperwork and pray that the involuntary hold serves useful for her. Inpatient admission is an important opportunity to rest from the stressors of outside obligations, time for introspective thought, development of insight into illness, and a safe environment to trial medications for stabilization.

In all this, I do leave room for curiosity, and between you and me, I'm personally pulling for something along the lines of alien abduction or alien nano-technology implants as being the root cause. Even a good governmental cover-up would prove to be so much more intriguing than watching someone crumble through disorders of psychiatric illness. Plus, it's probably easier to fight aliens and the pesky nanobots than to convince someone with delusional disorder that the only unwanted infiltrations in their body are those of faulty synapses and neurotransmitters, both adrift from their rightful course.

CHAPTER 8

Escaping Escobar

STEPHANIE

"Your daughter has schizophrenia," I told the woman.
"Oh, my God, anything but that," she replied. "Why couldn't she have leukemia or some other disease instead?"
"But if she had leukemia she might die," I pointed out. "Schizophrenia is a much more treatable disease."
The woman looked sadly at me, then down at the floor. She spoke softly. "I would still prefer that my daughter had leukemia."
—E. Fuller Torrey, M.D.

On day 3,545, I receive the information regarding my next psychiatric consult while the patient is simultaneously being tended to in the emergency department for self-inflicted wounds. These "self-inflicted bilateral lacerations" were most likely conceived to create a tributary for fast-moving blood, the typical target of their source being the radial artery deep within the wrist. Verbal and written accounts percolating from the emergency room suggest a picture of a bloody initial portrayal. Yet further and more detailed inspection displays relatively superficial lacerations, and imaging for determination of underlying tissue damage is negative. These wounds of less-than-lethal intent will, however, still require suturing to assist in healing and for the prevention of infection.

Stephanie is a 16-year-old female brought to the emergency department by police officers after authorities were alerted to a person endorsing suicidal ideations. According to family, the patient was contemplating cutting her wrist with a kitchen knife while acting "odd" and reporting delusions of paranoia with content of being hunted by the "drug cartels." When police responded, the patient was sliding her arms back and forth on barbed wire fencing in an attempt to cut her wrists. Per police reports, she initially struggled, refusing police intervention, but was quickly subdued.

I await medical clearance and allow the youth some time to settle into her new room. I make my way to the pediatric psychiatric unit. Oddly, to get to this small unit of the hospital, one must first make his or her way through the obstetrics and gynecological unit followed by the mother and baby unit. The journey through these areas always earns me peculiar looks as people seem to think I'm lost and blindly searching for the cafeteria. Not to mention when a man with tattoos, facial hair, and fashioned in scrubs walks through these units, you can almost taste the fear in the air from all the new parents carefully guarding their newborn gifts. I don't blame them; in fact, if I saw myself walking alone in the neonatal unit as I held my new and better version of myself, I too would stay vigilant to this odd-looking man's behaviors. Although settings such as this make me uneasy in my own skin, I still appreciate being the unorthodox and obvious variant regarding what a physician is expected to look like. Over time, I have grown to appreciate that being unique is a hell of a lot better existence than being simply alive as the standard representation of what others anticipate.

I finally make it out of my own head and to my destination. After a short knock, I enter the room I have been searching for and provide my usual introduction and pleasantries. I find whom I suspect to be my patient sitting upright in bed with what appears to be another high-school-aged girl seated beside her. Her friend's chair is pulled up to the bedside and the two look to be involved in some juicy adolescent gossip.

"Wow. This is a nice room. How's the food over here?" I remark in an effort to display a carefree attitude and that of diverted focus from the patient's potential expectation of oncoming judgement.

"It's good. I had chicken strips and fries for lunch. I'm a vegetarian, but I made an exception today."

At first glance, her affect and mannerisms are hardly indicative of a girl who only a few hours ago wished for death.

I look to the vegetarian connoisseur of chicken strips seated upright in the elevated hospital bed. "You must be Stephanie."

"That's me," she responds, providing a reactive and carefree smile.

I can immediately see she has full range of movement with both hands via the way she manipulates her beverage, carefully guiding the straw to her mouth with her dominant hand. She also displays the ability to flex her wrist to turn down the volume of the television using the remote control found on the side of her bed. This all suggests that, despite the gruesome tales from the ER staff, her wounds are grossly cosmetic. This is not to discount the severity of her attempt, but to simply provide insight into the underlying objective. For example, intent that is less than critical may be a sign of someone with intense inner turmoil begging to be noticed. A cry to not be weighed for the surface-level injury but for the formidable depth of underlying pain. The real danger is to lose focus from the patient's disposition that is pleading for help. If the patient feels this internal misery is not recognized secondary to a less-than-critical suicidal gesture, they may increase in acuteness, or overall potential for lethality, any future suicidal gestures to garner the attention equal to their suffering.

The pediatric floor at this hospital is the old obstetrics floor, and therefore all the rooms are much larger than the conventional. Each room is designed with ample space and extra chairs that fold into beds for guests. These rooms are adorned with upgraded, wooden accents wherever the standard white plastic would not suffice. There are large windows for stunning views of the mountains, with visibility reserved for only the clearest of days, however few they may be.

The overall sense of each room appears to be aimed at the feeling of being a sterile master bedroom. The extra presence of cherry-wood trim provides just enough influence to give the serenity of a lakeside cabin. I'm guessing these tender touches make the experience of pushing a ten-pound baby out of a vagina ever-more comforting. This clearly provides an ambiance ripe for birth and one that is much more peaceful than the ever-present hustling of screams and bells found on the other hospital floors, although one can surmise with high likelihood that this floor has had its historical share of screaming and wailing from women in the throes of labor, each expressing their hatred for the men who sit idly perched as helpless ornaments at the bedside. While she lies bearing the burden of such life-giving trauma, he remains fixed with his only purpose being that of a hand holder and motivational speaker.

I found all the deliveries that I scrubbed into during medical school to be traumatic to watch. In fact, while obviously less painful, I would be willing to guess that the spectators of birth are witness to much more vivid scenes of harsh nature in action than those unfortunate but brave women suffering through the process. I can attest; I have seen what I consider to be human atrocities during a cesarean section, watching as the obstetrician uses his gloved hands to tear and rip the layers of the female abdomen. A cruelty, better yet, a symbolic gateway, for innocence to be birthed into a world so similar in its essence. I would say I have been more comfortable assisting in a below-knee amputation or small bowel perforation than I ever was during a cesarean section.

Stephanie is now up and pacing around the room excitedly, or nervously, I can't quite tell. She and her friend spend some time exchanging glances from across the room as she intermittently giggles while adjusting every little thing she can get her hands on. This appears to be less of an impulse created by psychosis or mania and more of a joyful response to the attention she is now receiving.

I attempt to quiet her restless actions by being the calming influence this assessment requires. I find a seat at the circular wooden table in the corner of the room as my eye catches a checkerboard with pieces not yet in play. "Ah, I love checkers. Play me?"

"Sure!" She quickly takes the only other chair at the table and sits directly across from me.

I look at her friend. "It's really cool that you came here to support your friend." I look at Stephanie. "You are lucky to have such great friends."

"She's my cousin . . . well, and my friend." They again share a giggle.

I again look to her friend. "Do you mind if I chat with Stephanie for a little bit in private? I'll come and grab you when we are done." I make eye contact with the nurse who has followed me into the room to escort the girl out so that we can maintain some confidentiality. This affords Stephanie the privilege of answering my questions without fear of teenage judgement.

"Okay, black or red?" I ask.

"I'll be black."

"Okay, cool, I'm red."

I make the first move on the board and we begin, engaged in the slaughter of each other's pieces as we chat. One by one the pieces disappear, and I soon realize the score is unequivocally in my favor. I remind myself that I should allow her to win and to accomplish such in a subtle manner of gracious defeat. The last thing I figure a teen's fragile sense of self-worth needs is an ass kicking at a meaningless board game. As we play, I inject questions of great importance, yet with the tone of a curious friend.

"Dude, what happened? Why are you here?"

"I tried to kill myself," she responds, frighteningly unconcerned with the subject matter.

"How did you try to kill yourself?" I ask, without making eye contact as I pretend to be torn between my next move.

She prefers a display of sorts rather than a verbal response. She extends both arms at the elbows while resting her forearms on the table, and she motions to the large gauze bandages covering each wrist.

"Oh, man, that looks painful."

"Yeah," she replies.

"Why did you want to kill yourself?"

"I don't know." Shrugging her shoulders and staying focused on the game, she gives me no inclination to actually believe this, so I continue to cautiously pry.

"Well, I remember being a teenager. It sucked, and high school . . . I hated high school."

"Yeah, high school sucks, but I guess it isn't that bad."

"Is there anyone at school you want me to beat up for you?" I ask this to try find a circumstantial answer to the unsaid question regarding bullying.

She laughs. "No, it's pretty chill at my school."

"Okay, well, I'm going to be honest with you. I'm worried about you, and I'm sure your family is worried as well. Let's think about why you want to die. I can't imagine that's a good feeling to have. I mean, stuff has got to be pretty bad to want to end it all, you know?"

"Yeah. I don't know. I just feel like my family would be better off without me."

"What makes you say that?"

"I don't know. I guess I just feel like a burden."

I still wait to see some semblance of pain or heaviness in her expression. Surely, a congruent affect, with the severity of the current topic, would be one of depression or sadness. Yet, she appears unfazed.

I lessen my caution regarding direct questions. "Well, I know sometimes people get bullied at school or online. Either of those ever happen to you?"

"No, I'm pretty popular."

"Well, that's good." I make another move to break the questioning up a bit and to try further deescalating her guard. "Finally, I got one of yours!" I raise one arm up in celebration and smile to distract her. "I meet a lot of people your age going through some of the same feelings of wanting to end their life. A lot of times these guys or girls have been victimized. Sometimes someone has taken advantage of them or hurt them in some way. Has anything like that ever happened to you?"

"You mean like sexually?"

"Well, people can be hurt in many ways. Sexual abuse, physical abuse, verbal abuse."

She interrupts me. "No. That's never happened to me."

"Okay, good. I just needed to ask. Just know in the future if anything like that does happen, there will always be people out there to help you. Okay?"

"Okay," she responds, nodding her head.

I continue to press. "So how are you feeling after all this? I mean, do you wish you would have died or are you happy to be alive?"

"I'm okay either way, but I still want to kill myself."

"Well, I appreciate your honesty. I was told you were concerned people may be out to harm you. Do you still feel that way?"

"Not right now. Sometimes I catch people following me or sometimes I'll see the same car like three or four times drive down my street in a short amount of time. I don't know, it's weird. It's hard to explain. It's like a feeling."

"I get it, and you're right; sometimes feelings are hard to describe to others, especially when we don't truly understand them ourselves. Well, do you at least feel safe here?"

"I do," she replies, again focusing more on her next move than the question at hand.

Maybe that is her way to deflect the question. Maybe she is suffering from paranoia, or maybe someone really is after her. However, if I was a betting man, I'd say maybe, just maybe, she keeps the answers short and simple to keep me from picking apart the details of her story. Honestly, at this point, it doesn't matter to me if she hurt herself to get attention or if she truly wants to die. My only concern is her safety. There are countless graves filled with people who attempted suicide or engaged in impulsive behaviors, not with the intention of dying, but to draw attention to their inner conflicts or struggles. Many of those who accidentally succeeded in suicide just wanted attention or just wanted to be heard.

For now, I will make sure she gets the attention she desires, with the hope that she will find the help she needs. Some mental health professionals would hold onto the diagnostic idea of needing to quickly determine a diagnosis. I have no need for this, and I have no problem admitting it's too early to know. In this case, borderline personality disorder, which can present with intermittent micro-psychotic breaks, will remain on my differential, along with prodromal phase of schizophrenia, major depressive disorder with psychotic features, and numerous other potentials of diagnostic significance. For me, however, it is much too early to give anything but care. Labels will have to wait.

At this point, I have already decided her fate will be admission to a mental health facility. However, I go ahead and ask her opinion, providing the much-needed illusion that she is in control of her own destiny. "Are you cool with going to a mental health hospital for a little bit just so we can keep an eye on you and help you through this rough time you're having?"

"Yeah. I think that would be a good idea."

"Awesome! You made that nice and easy for me. I appreciate it."

She smiles. "No problem."

I set up my last piece for her to easily take, and with her victory, she gives me yet another smile. She likely knew I was making a lot of foolish moves on purpose, but sometimes just winning can bring joy, regardless of the road to the checkered flag. Our mind has a unique way of making us think we deserve things we didn't actually earn, and I use that neuro-idealism to my advantage today.

"Okay, you seriously kicked my butt. I'm the doctor; you are supposed to let me win."

She giggles again.

"Alright, I'm going to leave in shame now. I need to call your parents and chat with them and let them know what we decided. Is that cool?"

"Yeah, that's cool."

"Alright, Steph, I better get to work before I get in trouble. Rematch tomorrow?"

She laughs. "Heck yeah, but you better bring your 'A' game."

"Damn, look at you. I like it. Alright, I'll come by in the morning and bug you. Get some rest." I reach out my fist and she reciprocates in appropriate fist-bump fashion.

I exit the room and head over to the nurse's station. I turn to the nurse who I assume is currently in charge of Stephanie's care, since she is the one who followed me into the room. I ask for the parent's contact information and she quickly provides me with a sticky note of the information. I ring the only number provided, assuming her parents are still married. I reach Stephanie's biological father, who is indeed still married to her biological mother. A small win for my mini patient.

I first authenticate some of the information Stephanie provided during our board game, such as medical history, medications, both current and previous medication trials, and previous suicide attempts. I then try to grasp his overall feel for what is happening with his daughter, as well as address any questions or concerns he may have. What I uncover seems to be the prototypical middle-class family struggling to survive financially and emotionally, and seemingly doing a pretty good job at it. Of course, having your daughter persistently trying to harm herself won't win you any parent of the year awards, but those familiar with mental illness would understand these factors are often beyond parental influence or control. He and his wife seem to be legitimately concerned for their daughter and have been taking the appropriate steps to find her the help she requires.

The scariest realization for me when talking with him was his similar experience with her incongruent affect. For example, he reports that days before her most recent incident, all seemed fine and there was no indication of depression or suicidality. It had been a regular week with band practice after school and sleepovers with her friends. Nothing seemed out of the ordinary, and to his amazement, he actually felt as though she seemed happier than she had been in months. Then, without warning, she decided she was suicidal during the morning of the incident. This was after a cheerful family breakfast and as everyone was getting ready to partake in the normal weekend activities. This included attending a theme park for her younger brother's birthday, which she seemed quite enthusiastic about attending.

Her sudden change in outward display of behavior not only shocked him and his wife but it took away their small sense of confidence regarding knowing their own daughter. They are especially fearful of what she might do in the future, as they have no way to predict or even sense the oncoming storm in mentality their daughter shifts between. They feel defeated, and I assure them that we were admitting her to a pediatric mental health facility for stabilization and treatment. I also assure them that we will do everything in our power to help.

I hang up the phone, realizing that I share in the fear of what she may do. The worst part is that, with her intelligence, she will likely be able to maneuver an early discharge from the mental health hospital. Therefore, this admission will most likely do little to cure what aches inside her, but only time will tell.

I wasn't able to get that rematch in checkers as by the next morning she was already transferred to a mental health hospital that specialized in pediatrics about two hours south. With knowledge of her struggles, I have a feeling that, unfortunately, our paths will again cross. I'm certain we will share another board game in the near future, and this time I'll bring my "A" game.

CHAPTER 9

A Mother's Burden

JENNY

"Being a mother is learning about strengths you didn't know you had and dealing with fears you didn't know existed."
—Linda Wooten

Postpartum psychosis with ideations of infanticide thoroughly intrigues me, both in complexity and morality. The struggle to grasp such a state still escapes my full cognitive acceptance; however, its realization as a disease state is comprehensible.

A woman carries a baby for nine months. Within this time, she embraces everything she can to provide her baby a safe environment for growth. She is forced to suffer through sickness, nausea, cramping, and the physical and emotional toll afforded by intense hormonal alterations. She thinks little of herself as her body is taken over as a vessel for life, and with this abduction, often the youth of her figure is kidnapped by biological necessity. She confronts great levels of stress and lethargy with focus and selflessness believing her sacrifice as only secondary to a deeper meaning and purpose. With great courage, she then faces the final dowry of pain and suffering through the act of childbirth. Subsequently, and in triumph, she is bestowed with the ability to hold her progeny and revel in the gift she has created. As this new life is rested upon her chest, an organic union between mother and baby is born. A connection arisen, both created and guided by countless previous generations and thousands of years of innate necessity for the survival of species. An experience so natural that often we lose sight of its simplistically complicated splendor. Skin to skin, heartbeat to heartbeat, mother and child are now one in a lifelong journey encompassing an unbreakable bond.

She can now sigh in relief as her struggle has nourished and given bloom to a flourishing example of herself, both innocent and pure. A version of the self, without limits. A soul free of judgement who cares nothing for race, ethnicity, or class. A vessel without political views or preconceived notions, and free from cynicism and hate. A life unexperienced and with it a life untarnished. Hope abounds as the manifestation of our dreams and aspirations is now encompassed in the form of a better version from our own reflection.

As we find ourselves vulnerable in joy, lying upon the beach of possibilities, a disconcerting chill evolves on the back of our necks. We reluctantly look up, just in time to see the radiance across the sky dissipate as darkness descends rapidly and unexpectedly. A storm blunting the sun's life-giving rays has jolted our ideals and we now scramble to take stock of the situation descending upon us. Panic sets in as the tide quickly rises and we find ourselves struggling to remain above water. Our feet, only moments ago stable in the fine, warm sand, are now ripped from below as the undercurrent pulls our understanding out to sea. When the tide finally recedes, something else finds its way to shore. The mother that so recently was fixated on the care of her child, emerges from the squall, drenched in disorganization and unlike the woman she had come to know. She no longer wishes for motherhood nor does she feel a connection to the innocence that was laid upon her barren chest. She now, and in stark contrast, expresses a wish of finality, with intentions to end her newborn's life.

It is an intensely counterintuitive outcome from all natural, biological, and child-rearing standards but an outcome that is all too real. The origination of such symptoms is unclear; however, it's possible those same stressors that had assigned drive and focus, all for the purpose of growth and conservation of life, have also, and ever so slowly, taxed the brain's ability to suitably adapt and function. The mind's interpretation of this unfamiliar role may be construed as a labor of fear, panic, and paranoia. The individual's feelings of being overwhelmed may only further the brain's inability to acclimate through appropriate neurotransmission. The mind lies untethered to interpret such emotions as self-doubt, and within the loss of identity, there are few options other than to decimate this new inciting stressor.

It's day 3572, and I'm about to come face-to-face with postpartum psychosis. Jenny has been still for the past three hours, ever since consuming the cocktail I ordered for her earlier this morning. Per nursing reports, the patient had been banging her head against the wall in an attempt at self-harm.

In the mental health hospital, we attempt to remove all items that could be used in an attempted suicide or for purposes of self-mutilation. Often those patients suffering from suicidality are forced to smash their heads against walls and windows in an attempt to relieve the urges to end their life. Sometimes these acts are purely out of frustration or feelings of guilt. There's nothing quite like a little haloperidol, lorazepam, and Benadryl, all swiftly injected to a human's buttocks, to calm the senses and bring the opportunity for reality back onto the horizon. This particular cocktail is called a B-52, after the famous American Bomber, for multiple reasons, one being that it is typically dosed at 50mg of "B"enadryl, "5"mg of haloperidol, and "2"mg of lorazepam. Aside from the numerical coincidence, the outcome of the cocktail is even more relateable to the flying fortress of World War II simply because B-52, in a sense, carpet-bombs the brain to calm all perceptual disturbances, anxiety, and emotions. The intent is, of course, to aim for a particular region of the brain, but with windage and brain chemistry, the cocktail has a habit of causing collateral influences.

As the sedation effects of her B-52 wear off, Jenny sluggishly comes to, and in a much more manageable state than her previous form. Her eyelids appear heavy and only moments away from removing her from partial wakefulness. Her eyes close even further as she strains to ascertain clear sight, all from the distance of the restraint bed secured purposefully in the center of the seclusion room. It's a true padded-room, as depicted frequently in cinematic dramatizations of psychiatric mental health facilities like the 1975 comedic-drama *One Flew Over the Cuckoo's Nest.*

As I stand before her, I notice my feet sinking ever so slightly into the soft, blue-padded flooring, which causes a strange sense of unsteadiness. The walls are completely covered with a puffy mattress-like material, except now in the shade of desert tan. In the middle of this rather small room is a hospital bed, affixed with the same blue upholstery that covers the floor. This cradle of sanity is additionally adorned with four sturdy brackets affixed to the bed providing an area of anchoring for the soft restraints. These forgiving restrictions remain in place, currently subduing all four of her limbs. Although she remains sedated and basically chained to the bed in which she lies, I can't help but feel the need to engage her and maybe gain some knowledge into her suffering. Regardless of previous or current behaviors, seeing another human, or even an animal for that matter, subdued via shackles is painful to the soul.

Our first encounter provides very little usable information, forcing a decision to forgo further questioning at this moment of captive agreeability. I shall wait for a time of less acuity and increased stability so that I may attempt to piece together where things diverged from evolutionary design.

It takes another three hours before Jenny is ready to be set free and moved back to the comfort of her room.

"Hello, Jenny. I'm Dr. McLaughlin. We met this morning. Do you remember me?"

Jenny turns her head gently towards the direction of my voice, taking a moment to look me in the eyes. In lieu of a verbal response, she shakes her head, denying memory of our previous meeting.

"That's okay if you don't remember me; you were a little sleepy this morning. Can you tell me how you're feeling now?"

She answers in a blunted sense of incongruency. "Fine."

"Are you in any pain?"

"No."

"Okay, good. Now, I don't want to upset you or bother you too much, but I am trying to learn more about you. That way I can do everything in my power to help you. To do that, I have to ask a few questions. Is that okay?"

She gives minimal response and looks away. We play the same game frequently found in car dealerships during negotiations. Whoever talks first loses. Her eyes slowly fill with tears, lips trembling, as her fingernails began to gnaw against the sheet lining her bed. It's as if she has an image in her head that she wants to claw out. I can almost see the brain's betrayal and her frustration of being at odds with her own mind. It's like the soul is longing for the right actions, but the brain, and the mind's interpretation of such, continues to guide her movements and intentions.

Then she responds. Her reddened conjunctivae continue to pour down copious amounts of tears, her fingers already looking sore as she continues to scratch and pull against the cloth barrier. Her left wrist is still bandaged from a reported self-inflicted knife wound, appearing to have numerous amounts of aged bloodstains. A quick inspection of this area thankfully displays no fresh signs of bright-red blood implying reinjury.

"I put a pillow over my son's face. He just wouldn't stop crying. I didn't want to do it, but I felt pushed, or pulled, to do it. It's like I couldn't help it, and I wasn't strong enough to stop. There was this voice that just kept telling me to do it."

"What made you stop?" I ask.

"I heard a different voice yell out, 'Jenny!' Then I was able to gain some sense of control over my arms."

I sigh and nod my head. "I understand you must be under a lot of stress, and I also understand how difficult a newborn can be, as I have a son of my own. They are completely reliant on their mother for food, comfort, and everything else. I'm sure it's a lot to deal with."

"It is. It really is."

"Let's start with an easy question. First, what about having a new baby in the home is wonderful, and second, tell me what is not so wonderful."

"I want it back," she whispers.

"It?" I ask, pretending as though I have no idea what she is talking about and donning a rather perplexed look across my face. "Jenny," I say sternly, pausing after to garner her full attention. "What exactly do you want back?"

"Someone took my baby, I think. How do I know that this baby is mine? My baby wouldn't cry this much. My baby would be happy."

I refuse to let her pass on the complexity of the current situation with such a meek statement of misidentification. I realize her mind is searching for justification for the acts committed. I will not allow this to be the sole cause of her mental decompensation and inability to love her child. "Jenny, when babies are born, they are given medical ID bracelets matching the birth mother so things like what you are suggesting don't happen. So, do me a huge favor. From now on, let's assume the baby you took home is the same baby you gave life to. The beautiful baby that you conceived, carried, and gave birth to is the same baby now resting at your home, peacefully awaiting his mother's return. Now, please tell me what else is going on that is making this time so difficult for you."

"Not right now. I need to sleep."

"Okay, Jenny, I will let you relax for the rest of the day because you deserve it. I will come bug you tomorrow morning, okay?"

"Okay." She turns her head away from me while closing her eyes. I witness her hand slowly relax and the pressure of her fingernails release their burden. Maybe she just needed some comforting words to assure her that her baby is truly hers and to disrupt any delusions of her baby being switched. This is not to say what I told her is some unique notion or one not persistently presented to her by her husband. Time and time again, our loved ones can tell us something over and over, yet it isn't until a stranger with some sort of credentials utters the same phrase that it holds merit. It's the finicky nature of the mind to doubt the words of people we know wish us no harm and to validate the opinions of those who have nothing to lose by their honesty.

I don't know yet how to treat Jenny's condition, but I do know the brain is an interesting organ that sometimes needs complex medication or medical interventions, while other times simply needs some structure, relaxation, and a good night's sleep.

On day 3573, I find myself back in the rural mental health hospital. There is something comforting about seeing patients here as I know when I leave for the night, they have nurses and staff looking after them with all the tools of modern medicine at their disposal. There is a sense of ease knowing that if a patient's condition decompensates medically and becomes more than we can handle at our facility, it's only a short ambulance ride to the emergency room at the main hospital. The inpatient unit provides the added luxury, from my standpoint, of providing me the opportunity to see my patients daily. I remain ever aware of their condition, constantly assessing them for changes in symptoms or medication effectiveness and monitoring them for adverse effects. Oftentimes, while in the outpatient setting, I'm forced to worry about my patients, as they are left to their own accord without my watching eyes. I may prescribe a medication or change the dosing and then not see them again for a full four weeks. An entire month of not knowing can be uniquely daunting, anxiety-provoking, and sleep-depriving. Not here, though, not in this locked unit full of medical professionals. For now, I as well as Jenny, can rest comfortably and securely.

The first thing I do the next morning is call Jenny's husband and gather some collateral information regarding her past psychiatric history. I attempt to develop a timeline of events throughout her pregnancy and different symptoms he was privy to witness. From our conversation, he appears to be a loving and supportive husband and father, and it appears there have been road signs for her impending breakdown. To someone with experience in mental health, some of her road signs could be considered massive billboards with big, flashing neon lights, warning everyone around her of the danger to come. To those without experience, these are simply symptoms of something they cannot understand. It is so much easier to tell yourself that this phase or stage will end soon, and everything will be back to normal. It's much more difficult to see diverging roads of normalcy as indications of a path into darkness.

It wasn't until she was found in the kitchen, holding a large kitchen knife while staring out the kitchen window whispering to herself in conversation of pleading and deal-making, that the gravity of her illness was realized. As her husband slowly approached to relieve her of the knife, he noticed her left wrist had been cut and was bleeding quite profusely onto the kitchen floor. He asked her why. Jenny verbalized that just moments ago she almost killed their newborn son with a pillow. In shock, he does what he can to repress his anger towards her, fighting the genetically predetermined will to neutralize any threat to his offspring. In a display of higher brain functioning, he tends to her fragile state while carefully removing the knife from her hand. As he stood wrapping a towel around his wife's self-inflicted attempt at suicide, he recalls to me that he realized he could no longer hide from the truth of her illness. At this time, he called 911 while applying pressure, doing his best to slow the bleeding until the ambulance arrived.

In that moment, as he held a cloth to her intention to die, he heard his son cry in the other room. He recalls a strange feeling of being soothed by his son's crying, as it was a sign that he was indeed alive, a relief to his innermost fear. I commend him for his quick action. I also explain to him the reason for her admission, just in case he had not heard the official reasoning. I also do my best to provide dictation of something that could be considered as a plan. I reveal the diagnosis, or the diagnosis I believe to be accurate, as I have checked all labs and ruled out most organic causes. Of course, there could be some rare etiology underlying these outward symptoms of devastation, which is something we call a "zebra," but usually the sound of hooves is just a horse.

I explain that patients with postpartum psychosis are at an increased risk of suicide, neglect for their baby, as well as the potential for infanticide. I express my concern for the possibility of a suicide attempt with possible completion if she is not fully stabilized prior to release. There is also a chance that her underlying condition will show its face as a diagnosis of bipolar disorder in the future, but as I expressed, this can be attended to if it arises. With these increased risks, even after acute stability is achieved and discharge is granted, the patient should not immediately be left alone with the child for some time and must be monitored closely for reoccurrence of symptoms.

I inform him that, in my opinion, stabilization using medications should be maintained for a minimum of 12 months secondary to the severity of her current and recent states. If after 12 months there is a consensus, then a gradual dosage taper and even possible complete discontinuation may be attempted if, and only if, performed under the strict observation of an outpatient psychiatrist. It may be a little early for such a statement, but a doctor's perspective involving future resolution does wonders to lead the patient and their families to a positive outlook. One would be amazed at the benefits and power of optimism and confidence in the face of vulnerability. The mind-body connection is a powerful and often untapped resource in the course of recovery from any illness.

Once I'm done explaining all this, he shares a fact for which I was absolutely unaware. "I think this is just a really stressful time for Jenny, especially after we lost our first baby to SIDS."

It is with great embarrassment that I admit it wasn't until I was in my car driving home that evening that I theorized a potential connection. The loss of their first baby to a disorder, free of an agreed-upon cause, in a patient suffering currently from symptoms of postpartum psychosis provides a theory of association without any great need for thought. I often wonder why I never made the connection immediately, overlooking the potential for relationship among two distinct incidents that no longer appear to be singular. The interesting thing is the other resident psychiatrist who was shadowing my interview that day also made no connection until I brought it up to him later that night during a call of panic. Maybe we were both too fixated on the gravity of the situation before us that we could not look behind it for historical significance. Although this theory that I had in such an untimely manner was most likely having properties free of proof, I feel it is the essential duty of a psychiatrist to quickly make potential linkages when presented with them. I guess there is an art to learning from life's mistakes and failures, and if this holds true, then I must be the Van Gogh of medical professionals.

Unfortunately, Jenny was not able to discern the warnings, and she nearly ended the life of her child. The mind has a tricky way of normalizing the brain to odd occurrences. Sometimes the mind just fills in the gaps of ridiculous notions to simplify their probability. It is much simpler and comforting for the mind to believe everything is normal than to break the status quo for the option that we are losing our hold on reality. Her husband confirmed the evidence of a stressed and struggling brain, a brain ultimately responsible for the generation of emotional lability, delusions, and hallucinations. Fortunately, the baby and the mother are both currently safe, so not all is lost. I assure the husband prior to the end of our call that with proper medication, stress-management, family presence to decrease the burden of her duties, and therapy, she will recover and return to the loving wife and mother he knows so well.

After the call, I go talk to Jenny. I find her in the community room, which houses a localized television, couches, and tables used for snack and art time. She is wearing her blue scrubs, with a white blanket over her shoulders like a shawl. Completing the outfit are the yellow hospital socks with the white texture on the bottoms to provide grip. Her hair appears combed, yet still partially wet from a likely morning shower. She is standing quietly, looking out the window and onto the central courtyard grass. I hope she is thinking of her son and all the games they will play in the grass. I hope she is picturing her and her husband swinging their son up with his legs gliding through the air, and every time his little shoes touch the ground he is heard shouting out, "Again, again," followed with laughter as both parents look to each with the glow of happiness only a child can bring.

"Good morning, Jenny," I say quietly as I approach her. "Can we chat for just a little bit?"

"Sure."

"I'm Dr. McLaughlin. I am a resident psychiatrist here. Do you remember me?"

"I do. We met yesterday."

"Great. So how did you sleep last night?"

"I slept good, like all night."

"It's pretty outside, isn't it? Would you like to chat outside?"

"Okay."

The mental hospital is an older building shaded by trees with large walls encasing the structure in an almost perfect square. One side of the complex is a locked unit housing male and female patients with less-severe psychiatric acuity, such as those without intentions of suicide or homicide. This unit I call "the petting zoo," with obvious implications of being harmless except some transmissible diseases as any petting zoo provides. The other side is a different animal altogether. Women and men are housed in separated and locked units. This I call the "pink pit" or "blue pit," depending if you find yourself on the female or male side. This name reflects the obvious danger these units deliver.

In the middle is a large, grassed area, "the courtyard," which all the units are connected to through their own access doors. Each unit is also affixed with multiple barred windows facing into this same courtyard should you wish to squint through the haze of tempered glass to garner stunning views of grass growing. Here the patients have the opportunity to exercise, throw frisbees, and play catch with a football. Some prefer to just sit and tan; others partake in some form of interpretive dance, which is always original and off-key to the music in the background. Music is provided by the unit's circa-1980, silver, dual-speaker boombox. The time in this courtyard is always a guilt-provoking joy to watch, as the medications slow down reaction times leading to a plethora of "oh shit" moments that only objects thrown or kicked to one another can provide.

I open the door to the courtyard, and we sit at the first of many tables. The table is riddled with small holes throughout, purposefully manufactured in a way to give all fluids, regardless of source, clear access to fall through to the floor. She is seated at the bench closest to the door, and I am sitting directly across from her.

We start in typical fashion, talking about the weather, where she lives, where she grew up, school, and her life in general as a child and teenager. I oddly find no red flags. She has no previous trauma I can discover, no history of suicidality, and no recounts indicative of prior psychosis. She is without previous psychiatric history, and I find no genetic predisposition as her family history is clear. From all accounts, she was just your normal happy woman, until she wasn't.

Aside from her recent episode of psychosis, Jenny appeared to have a natural history as a sweet and caring individual—up until the moment she attempted to murder an innocent child.

I listen attentively as she explains the conditions of her psychosis from its inception.

It has been three days since Jenny's arrival and things have begun to improve. Her wrist is nearly healed, and I am able to elicit a smile today, and best of all, I have the pleasure of removing her stitches.

The psychiatrist is allotted very little occasion to perform procedures, so even something as mundane as suture removal becomes a priority when the opportunity arises. We, like other physicians, go through the same medical school and the same rotations. We participate in surgeries, perform physical exams, stitch lacerations, and, of course, dissect, so it is with the occasional jealousy that I pass a bustling emergency room or surgical operation wishing I could scrub in and get my hands dirty. Maybe it is a good thing, though, as the last time psychiatrists took to the scalpel, they found themselves driving spikes into the brain, lobotomizing patients to ascertain calm dispositions in the face of psychosis.

As I remove the bandage to expose the area, I take a moment to express my thankfulness to her that she did not get a chance to complete her act. I do this, not only because I care, but also to see if she agrees or refers to a sense of wishing it would have been completed. She also created a horizontal laceration on the wrist, which is much too shallow to do the job before being discovered by a family member. Maybe she wasn't actually trying to end her life; maybe she was self-inflicting punishment for what had transpired earlier in the day. Maybe realizing a sense of willingness to end the life of your child sends a self-destruct impulse to the brain in a biological act to save your genetic progeny. It is no different from someone living in a ball of hurt mixed with delusion, and her every problem stemmed from being unable to accept the reality of her current situation.

She details recently being plagued with auditory hallucinations of hearing a child counting numbers and singing lullabies when it was obvious it could not have been her newborn. She endorsed the experiences of hearing voices conversating seemingly to each other, voices being derogatory by telling her she is a horrible mother, and a voice telling her to kill her baby and herself. What she described as being most distressing was hearing a baby cry constantly, and when she would check her baby, he would be sound asleep. Even with her baby asleep, the crying would continue.

"Sometimes when the crying wouldn't stop, I'd go to his crib and fight back the want to shake him till the crying stopped, even if he wasn't the source. It was like the crying was permanently in my head. It was so strange. It's hard to describe. Sometimes I would feel like my baby had been swapped, even though my husband never left his side in the hospital. Sometimes I would think the crying baby I was hearing was my baby that had been stolen from me. This only made me even more upset with the baby in the crib next to my bed. I know I must sound crazy. Well, obviously I'm crazy, look where I'm at." She looks at me while nervously laughing.

I return a sincere yet reserved smile. "Well, you're certainly not crazy. Stressed and overwhelmed? Yes, but not crazy."

"My expectations were so high. I was so excited when I brought him home, but then I remember being utterly terrified. I remember putting him in the car at the hospital and thinking, 'Oh my God, how am I going to do this? I have no idea what I'm doing.' It felt like too much."

"How did you get through that initial phase with your baby?" I ask.

"In the beginning, I had my mother and other family members always coming by and helping out. Slowly, as the weeks went by, I guess the novelty of the baby wore off and people came by less and less. Even my own mother stopped helping me as much."

"I bet she felt like you were doing a great job and probably didn't want to impose."

"Yeah, that's probably true. I guess I just wish when things started happening that I would have realized what was going on and asked for help. Even my husband had no idea until the end, at least I don't think he did."

We continue on for another twenty minutes, going over what occurred week by week. She told me of suffering from delusions of paranoia, thinking the voices were a trick to drive her crazy and all a ploy of the individuals who switched her baby. She often felt like she was being watched by these same individuals and would take steps to check her home for hidden cameras and hidden voice recorders.

I attempt some greater-than-surface-level retrospection as she appears to have appropriate insight into the occurrences. I hope this insight will impart proof merely by the lack of validity for which she believed to be truth. Once plagued by paranoia, she appears to slowly display increased resolution of such and an overall sense of lessened anxiety. Over time, Jenny continues to report persistent auditory hallucinations, but slowly the content became less intrusive with decreased influence over her attention. She begins to re-wire her brain through repetitive guidance and self-coping mechanisms. As her brain begins to lose its hold for destruction, her mind follows with lessened coercion of thoughts. As the days progress, she continues to improve.

It was at this time, the time close to achieving her baseline level of functioning, that she inquires regarding a designation of her diagnosis.

"Can you tell me about my diagnosis? I mean, what do you think is wrong with me?"

"Well, the good news is nothing is wrong with you. You had a difficult time recently, most likely due to stress, but it could happen to anyone. If we wanted to name it, I'd say you had an episode of postpartum psychosis. That's basically saying that because of childbirth, changes in hormones, and the tons of stress on you, your mind had difficulty processing everything. Your thoughts became confused and you had a brief moment of impaired reality. Now, as you can tell, you are getting better and soon you will be back to your old self."

I remember she responded with something that resonates in the lack of complete education we provide to women who become pregnant about what to expect psychiatrically during the months of pregnancy and after delivery. She said, "Postpartum psychosis? I have never heard of that. I didn't even know it was a thing."

It takes another five days before Jenny's symptoms are resolved to the extent that I feel comfortable enough to send her home. My comfort, however, will be forever lying upon a fault-line of concern, never truly feeling the ground solid below me, as a tremor of fear and doubt will be present whenever I think about her. I pray that she finds resolution in all that ails her, and I hope her illness is overshadowed by the love and joy of her newborn baby. I have learned what countless before me already hold to be true, that there is no greater love than that of a parent for their child. It is through the love for our children that we often find the true meaning of life.

After a primary episode of postpartum psychosis, about a third of women will recover and suffer no further issues throughout life. The remaining two-thirds of women will have episodes outside the perinatal period, usually within the bipolar spectrum. The exact mechanism of onset is unknown yet may be related to the physiological changes after birth caused by hormonal and immune system alterations. The added stress and change in sleep patterns may be all that is required to precipitate postpartum psychosis in genetically vulnerable women. Regardless of the cause, inpatient care is usually required to ensure safety, complete the diagnostic evaluation, and to appropriately initiate treatment. The main reason for inpatient admission, however, is to provide safety to both the newborn and the mother. The relapse risk after a subsequent pregnancy for women with isolated postpartum psychoses is about 30%. Strategies for prevention of postpartum psychosis in someone with a history of such include providing prophylaxis mood stabilizers immediately postpartum, such as lithium or antipsychotics, along with proactive safety protocols and stress reduction techniques.

Psychosis after childbirth is a psychiatric emergency with elevated risks for suicide and infanticide. Immediate steps should be taken to provide safety. Don't suffer in silence and be not afraid of the stigma of mental illness. There is truly nothing to be ashamed of. Psychiatric illness is an illness of the brain and no different than any other illness of any other organ. If you or someone you know is suffering, please reach out for help.

CHAPTER 10

For the Love of Pain

SYLVIA

"When trained to feel nothing but pain,
the mind will crookedly search for such."
—PM

Is it because they have no respect for life that some men find it necessary to assault, abuse, and take advantage of women? Are these men who are committing daily atrocities heartless, soulless, or simply too lost in their cowardly ways to confront a more suitable opponent? Is empowerment fed by the quickening pulse of your victim, a victim overcome by fear, wondering if this is how their story ends? Often these men—or should we say dastardly invertebrates with testicles—find a sense of fulfilling power in overcoming the will of someone less able to defend themselves.

Maybe this isn't the best time to document the story of Sylvia. Just this morning, I read in my newsfeed about the tragic story of a female jogger in New York City who was overcome, beaten, and strangled to death. Reports reflect multiple defense wounds indicating she fought desperately for her life, only to have it stolen from her. After death, her attacker further desecrated the sanctity of life and discarded her naked, lifeless body in weeds and soot.

My own pulse quickens whenever I realize the evil that all men possess—a notion that any man can descend to depravity should the right stimulus arise. I believe we are all capable of atrocities under the right circumstances, while at the same time, each has a possibility of greatness. This potential, however, is often left uncovered and spoiled in blood among the evil deeds we have buried upon this opportunity. It truly is so much easier to destroy and cover the world in the same darkness that shadows your heart than to allow yourself the ability to grow from life's sufferings and misfortunes. It is altogether simpler to allow rejection and anger to spill over into life. This flood overtakes the actions required to fill the sandbags needed to hold the tide back. With each surge of adversity, a much-needed opportunity for insight, often as single elements of knowledge, are lost from each leak left untended.

On day 3651, I wake up to find myself to be a third-year resident. I'm not sure of the repercussions of such a title, as I don't feel particularly smarter or taller than the previous night. Still, I feel unprepared for the career path I chose even with ten years of study under my belt. Maybe soon I will reflect on how impressionable and naïve I was just a mere eight hours before my new title as an upperclassman. I go to put my pants on and realize it feels like it did the day before. I look at my new self in the mirror and, unfortunately, find myself no greater in stature or looks. One thing that will change is the location of my experiences. I say goodbye to the hallows of madness for the next 12 months, aside from nightly call shifts. I will be spending the upcoming continuum of 365 days in outpatient clinics.

This new setting provides for a quick lesson, as on day one I learn the fear of working with patients who get to leave you after an evaluation. They simply walk out, taking their prescriptions home and trying out whatever cocktail they have been prescribed. It is much different than the constancy of the inpatient realm with its many cameras and vigilant staff keeping an eye over the flock while you sleep. No longer having an ever-present sentinel of safety, I will now find myself in constant worry. "Did I choose the correct medication? What if I'm not there and they have side effects? Did I go over all the possible adverse events they should be aware of?"

These concerns will grow to linger, interrupting countless nights of sleep. I will become accustomed to awakenings covered in sweat, questioning myself. *Did I go over suicide precautions? Did we put in an appropriate crisis plan? Wait, what if they hurt themselves anyway? Maybe I could just call each patient every night to check on them. Is that even allowed? No, of course not.*

In order to be the physician my patients need; I put on my big boy pants and prepare for the trek to become a functionally competent outpatient psychiatrist. I'm one who would rather just jump in the deep end and figure it out while other more composed minds find themselves slowly wading in the shallow end of the pool analyzing every possible outcome.

After a long drive to an even more desolate part of the already sparse county, I find my office nestled amongst other unmarked buildings. Inside, I begin to decorate this new dwelling to my liking, knowing I will be spending countless hours within these four walls over the next year. My first order of business, as in any psychiatric office, is to remove all objects that could be used against me.

I'm handed a blue paper chart, as thin as such a chart would be if just removed from its box. I flip open the cover to examine my first patient's details only to find a blank state of historical data. No previous notes and no previous medications. No labs and no sign of a referral sheet from the patient's primary care doctor detailing the reason for our appointment. I head down the hallway from the cave I shall now refer to as my office. I open up the door to the waiting room of this newly appreciated and quaint outpatient psychiatric office, which is located in the absolute middle of nowhere. Upon hearing her name, Sylvia is prompted to carefully rise from her seat, with no quick movements and certainly without obvious intention to rush into her psychiatric evaluation.

She is a thin woman, partly balding or simply with very thin hair. She appears much older than her stated age of 45. I can tell her story, even before speaking with her, by her gait and lack of eye contact. Her height is just respectfully clear of five feet. Her shoulders seem to dictate a despondent layer of stress, torture, and defeat, much like an animal who has known nothing but pain and fear, holding its head and shoulders in a position of learned helplessness. I can tell she bears a visible burden of some unknown trauma.

I greet her with a hello and introduce myself. Little reaction is reciprocated by her, other than a poor attempt at a smile. She walks past me and towards the interview rooms, stepping ever so lightly. Each movement is purposeful in its progression towards gaining the inertia needed to carry her forward. Her gait appears as if she is walking barefoot on concrete on a hot summer afternoon.

Her steppage actually reminds me of the experience I had at my apartment pool only two days earlier. It was 105 degrees and the concrete surrounding the pool would actually burn the soles of your feet as you walked. Even just the short distance from the pool chairs to the quenching waters was a fiery trek across a teppanyaki grill. Sylvia reminds me of my son, as he would quickly tiptoe on the concrete whenever he exited the pool. Of course, this tiptoeing was only temporary and just until he reached the appropriate distance, only to sprint for another jump directly back into the pool, all while screaming, "Dad! Watch this!"

As we walk down the hallway, I say little, other than to direct her to the last room on the left. You can almost feel the depression, as if an emotion can have mass. These are the patients that are very difficult for me as I can almost sense the blooming sadness in my own personality. My persistent attempts to maintain a pleasurable and present demeanor begin to diminish, blunted by the grey cloud of hopelessness tugging at my shirt.

She walks noticeably slower than I am used to, so I intentionally take shorter strides, realizing how difficult it is to walk at the pace of most people, especially those without a sense of confidence in purpose. The speed of stride that medical professionals' traverse is a strange thing. Every attending I have had up to this point has been a fast walker and an even faster talker. Each doctor is seemingly guided by a persistent and heavy push forward from one patient to the next. In the early morning hours of my training, I would often wonder what the purpose of the morning rush was and how it factored into patient care. I remember thinking during my first year in the main hospital that there must be a reason behind such a hurried pace. Also, why the hell are we bothering them so early in the damn morning? Are medical symptoms at a heightened state in the hours before the sun rises above the horizon? Do the symptoms swim to the surface during the cool morning dew to feed, only to sink to the cold depths when touched with the warmth of sunlight? Maybe doctors are just sadistic in their militaristic training, with an unwritten rule of furthering the pain and suffering to their impressionable students, mimicking the tortuous path they themselves once faced.

As she carefully enters the exam room, I notice initial signs of a blunted affect, otherwise described as a reduction in emotional expressiveness, but I shouldn't be so quick to judge as I have yet to distinguish the underlying etiology related to her display of emotional reduction. She cares little for my observations and internal dialogue as she slowly settles into the chair across from my desk. Her lack of outward expression suggests no sense of distress, while at the same time, there is no indication of joy. She appears to just be present—present in a life that possibly didn't align with the one she had hoped for as a young girl.

Before I get a chance to sit down, she interrupts my momentum. I witness her looking down at her feet as they dangle off a chair that is much too tall for such a small woman. It is at this moment that she provides her first vocalization, a monotone statement with a most troublesome content. She doesn't raise her head to encounter my eyes and makes no alteration in her vocal inflection. She simply gazes at her feet and announces, "I want to show you something."

This is never something you want to hear from a psychiatric patient, especially while alone in the interview room. I slowly respond, "Okay," an action of non-committal to the upcoming follow-up statement she is about to share with me. I quickly glance in the direction of the door. Once assured the door is propped open with the appropriate stopper, I find myself descending cautiously into my own chair. It should be noted that this outpatient door stopper was created with such a purpose. Its plastic construction, appropriate angle, and floor-gripping bottom was quite the step up from the trash can I used in its place while on the inpatient unit. I gather my composure, waiting for a response as I prompt her, "What is it that you want me to see?" I am ready to give the request to stop should I feel it becomes inappropriate and needing the escort of a female nurse.

"I want to show you what I did to my toes."

A sense of relief comes over me knowing how badly that could have gone. Knowing the many parts of the human body that I am not keen on examining, at least not in this setting, makes anything to do with toes all the more bearable.

She slowly removes her worn tan shoes. I use the term of shoe lightly as they are more indicative of sandals with a strap to maintain placement and coverage. She slowly removes each shoe, putting on display her sockless, naked feet, when I notice something. It's not so much as what is present but what is lacking: a foot, or should I say a toe, without a toenail. The only thing worse than one bloody and mangled toe without a toenail is . . . you guessed it, ten bloody and mangled toes without toenails. You never realize that such an innocuous body part could produce such a strange and disturbing sight in its absence. I'm not sure if Darwin would agree, but I think the reason for toenails is because they simply look a hell of a lot better than toes without. I think it is highly possible that a group of well-adapted, prehistoric humans may have had absent toenails and, because of such, had limited breeding possibilities. This may have led to humans with this trait to slowly die off from a lack of willing participants in copulation.

"How did you do such a thing to your toes?" I ask, even before I have the time for a proper introduction.

"What do you mean?" she replies.

Attempting to clarify my question, I respond, "Well, what did you use to do such a thing?"

With a slight hint of almost pleasure, she responds, "I did it myself. I used my hands and slowly tore them off one by one."

Most likely looking more perplexed than concerned I continue to search for meaning. "Why would you do such a thing?"

She pauses, displaying some emotional response as she appears anxious to provide more detail than she has likely grown accustomed to sharing. "I like the pain; it feels good. I like to see the blood—the more the better. The voices tell me to do it. I can't help it. They tell me to do all types of things."

I make note of the auditory hallucinations reference; however, I attempt to stay focused on exploring one symptom at a time. "Tell me more about the sensation of pain and how it makes you feel."

"It's a relief. It's like when I cut myself. It's a feeling of released frustration." She continues on and, surprisingly, provides details without the necessity of prompting. "It's the only time I feel alive. Pain is the only emotion I know, the only emotion that reminds me I'm not dead."

"Tell me, how old were you when you started having the urge to hurt yourself?"

She lingers for seconds, possibly pondering or deep in thought, trying to remember where it all began. She begins to tell a story of finding her first release of frustration with cutting. "I went into the bathroom with a razor blade. I had the intention of ending my life. I chickened out, though. I was so pissed at myself for being weak that I started to cut my forearm with the blade, and you know what? I liked it; it felt good. Watching the blood running down my arms and pooling on the floor showed me that I could hurt someone and maybe I could defend myself. I felt like I had power. I would now bleed and feel pain when I chose, not when others chose it for me. From there it just got worse, and I was cutting every day. I had to start cutting on my upper thighs because people were starting to notice the cuts and scars on my arms."

As I sit in shock, I find myself alone in the setting of congruence with such a painful memory. There are no tears, no emotional response, just the detailing of a story of self-mutilation secondary to physical, emotional, and sexual abuse with no emotions displayed.

This type of behavior honestly doesn't strike me as odd, as I have found self-harm to be quite common, at least in my field of work. Reports suggest one in twelve teens, mostly girls, self-harm, and ten percent of them continue to deliberately harm themselves well into young adulthood. Many of these teens need help but are afraid to ask for it. One possible reason for their reluctance is the stigma associated with self-harming behavior and mental health in general. They fear that people will think they are crazy or trying to kill themselves. They fear they will be locked up and overly medicated. The stigma forces them to hide from help, holding the secrets inside, all while they sit against the locked bathroom door trying to feel some sort of release and relief from the agony inside. This deliberate self-harm is a way of expressing and managing anxiety, sadness, shame, and anger. It may also provide a temporary escape from emotional pain. This tactic may bring a sense of momentary relief, but the emotions often return with an increase in severity afterward, requiring more frequent and severe self-induced lacerations.

"I really appreciate you sharing this with me. It sounds like you have been suffering for a long time." I try to offer some consolation from the discomfort in telling a stranger your deepest and darkest secrets.

"Just know that any time you want to stop the interview, we can. Just please let me know. I realize this must be hard to talk about." I do this to afford her the ability to pull back on her disclosures. I give her the chance to say no if she does not feel like exploring her history with me any further at this time. It's a feeble attempt at allowing her to display some sense of control in her life. "Can we talk about the voices?"

She replies rather quickly, "What do you want to know?"

"Well, first of all, when did they start?"

"Oh, I have always heard voices." Making no eye contact, she focuses her gaze on the blank wall in front of her. Careful in her admission, she gives a vague answer in an attempt to simply move forward in the interview. I paternalistically don't allow for this comfort, at least not yet. If we move forward, her past becomes more confusing for her in its course. This is not uncommon as many people have difficulty in answering questions regarding time and initiation of symptoms. It's not something people usually think of, and therefore, it is my job to jostle the memory.

"So . . . for the last ten years?" I ask, hoping to give her a sense of the detail I'm searching for with my question.

"No. Since I was a kid."

I continue to pry. "Did it start before high school?"

"Oh yeah." She pauses as she gathers the strength to admit to me, and herself, of the long journey of suffering on a road paved with abuse and neglect. She begins to divulge more information, knowing that I'm going to continue to pester her should she continue to provide vague answers. "I was probably six or seven."

"Wow, that's young. You know, some children may begin to lose touch with reality after a traumatic event. Some may even begin to hear voices."

She again looks down at her toes. "My father and my brother."

"What about them? Did they hurt you?"

"My dad would come in at night after my mother fell asleep and he would rape me. Then, as my older brother became of age, he would do the same thing to me. It was like he learned from my dad that it was okay to force themselves onto me whenever they pleased."

"My God. I am so truly sorry that you had to suffer from that and suffer alone. You must have been a very strong girl to survive."

This conversation continues and leads to topics and details of the most horrific variety. Some are so horrifying that I have decided to not describe such offenses or place the actions of sickening men into printed word on pages. Their acts deserve nothing less than contempt and utter absence from written history.

Upon further exploration into her historical course of events, we find that Sylvia's voices appeared to coincide with the traumatic beginnings she faced alone, with initiation of psychosis occurring just after her seventh birthday. Her mother would not believe her and would often punish Sylvia for perpetuating such "lies." Her mother was possibly scared of her husband just as much as Sylvia feared his presence. It's also quite possible her mother would not allow herself to believe, because if she did, shame would fall upon their family and with it an assumption of guilt that she was not able to protect her daughter. It may simply have been a complete lack of situational awareness, an aloof presence, not able to engage in the reality before her.

Nonetheless, Sylvia's nightly incestuous encounters continued, and with it, the voices began to further along the suffering. She described these auditory hallucinations as derogatory in content. Often, she would be told by these voices that it was her fault and she deserved it; sometimes the voices would even give her commands to harm or kill herself. These voices would continue throughout her life, and Sylvia would begin to give credence to such statements, allowing her sanity to diminish with every admission of guilt. With this internal struggle of guilt, she began to lose focus in school and made no effort to make friends. She was forced to a course of isolation and felt her only self-worth was related to abuse.

With this came the depression, and it would have been quite easy to diagnose her with major depressive disorder with psychotic features until the context of persistent, unrelenting, and non-episodic psychosis was clarified. This designation was from the admission that although not constant, the voices did not initiate or coincide with an increased frequency or severity during times of severe depressive declines in mood.

Another possible diagnosis was that of schizoaffective disorder, depressed type; however, due to the unrelenting nature of her psychosis, a diagnosis of schizophrenia was preferred as the current working primary diagnosis. We must remember that patients with schizophrenia can often present with depressive symptoms, but this may also be misconstrued and related to the negative symptoms that are quite present in schizophrenia.

Due to her ever-present anxious predisposition in a multitude of situations, a secondary diagnosis of generalized anxiety disorder (GAD) could also be presumed, as well as a final and tertiary diagnosis of PTSD. This is because she would avoid situations that reminded her of her early years as well as persistent flashbacks of traumatic events, often so intense they would awaken her from slumber. It makes sense that a child in such a traumatic situation, alone and afraid with no one to turn to, would eventually blame herself for the pain and torture she was enduring. It is a way for the immature mind to cope with unfortunate events, a coping mechanism from a broken mind, severed from reality, and coupled with guilt. No one ever came to rescue her, and because of such, she was forced to inadvertently search in other men for the abuse she had only known.

Silvia was once someone's daughter, someone's sister. She was once a young girl who looked to the world as a place of wonderment. I can imagine her as the child who would run down the stairs on Christmas morning, just hoping to see her new bike posted under the tree as a gift from Santa Claus and his helpers. She checks on the plate of cookies and milk to find only crumbs and an empty glass, all further proof of his most recent presence.

Then one day, her world is smashed as the men in her life, the men she loved and relied upon, decided to steal her innocence for their own selfish sexual pleasures, filling the breach of trust with pain, confusion, and deceit. Had she only grown up with a different father, she may never have needed to schedule an appointment with me. Maybe we would have met in other circumstances. Maybe I would have commissioned her for assistance as a lawyer or accountant. Maybe we could have become close friends and confidants. Unfortunately, life is not always as we hope and is sometimes just what we are left to piece together. Sometimes there isn't enough left to build, and sometimes the mind becomes shattered.

Schizophrenia is a non-conforming beast. Those afflicted with such may have a genetic predisposition for it. It is an illness that may never arrive. Often, however, it is with the seeds of trauma that the illness takes root, growing out of control until it starves your future hopes and dreams of life. It is in this trauma that genetic predisposition is activated. Awakened from its slumber, it gives way to a lifetime cascade of mental illness. It is as if the mind reaches the point where it can no longer stand the struggle, and it fragments into its many pieces. The pieces are attached by nothing but misfires, all leading to distortions in perceived reality.

With the length of time and the severity of her symptoms, Sylvia clearly meets the diagnosis of schizophrenia. With this diagnosis comes a slow decline in functionality of the singular self. The strings of reality begin to dissolve, and the brain begins to lose preserved mass. Often those suffering from chronic schizophrenia have severe cognitive decline at a much earlier age than expected, only further complicating their struggles. This dementia, which arises from schizophrenia, is often analogous to dementia of other sources, leaving patients besieged both from lost memories and an even greater loss of function.

Sylvia continues to see me over the next year, and we become rather close. My goal in every appointment is simply to make her smile. Often successful, we make great strides in erecting the confidence and strength needed to build self-worth and self-respect. Like so many before her, she has a history of dating abusive men no different than her father. These relationships further cemented the course of struggle she was forced to travel upon. We spend many hours not only finding drive and purpose in life but also in recognition of destructive patterns of behavior.

I like to follow a rule that trauma should be explored once, and only once. Realization that it will not change, and it will not be explained, can add wonders to a sense of acceptance. She does well with this approach and flourishes in self-confidence over the months to come. So great is our progress that we are able to devise a strategy to safely remove her body from her current situation of persistent beatings and emotional abuse. She would slowly put money away, awaiting to have the funds to move out on her own. Her husband was never the wiser to our plan and knew not of what was in store. He most likely could not imagine his meek wife would build a sense of worth and harvest the confidence to stand up to him. He would need a new punching bag because this one was going to start punching back. That's exactly how I wanted her.

I couldn't have been prouder than when I realized she felt powerful and, better yet, capable. She began to like herself again, and with it, she learned to love herself. Loving ourselves is what keeps us searching for what we deserve. It is in Sylvia that I reflect on some of the greatest moments in residency: the moments spent watching women slowly take their lives back and slowly becoming the leaders of the own destiny as they were meant to be.

With patients such as Sylvia, the first order of business is to give therapeutic interventions regarding management of emotions as well as coping strategies and alternative methods of painful stimuli. Such patients often benefit from snapping a rubber band on their wrist when feeling the need to self-harm. Some will hold ice in their bare hand until it becomes painful. These are all better options than those related to self-induced bodily lacerations. Also, of key importance is that of psychopharmacology to address the underlying mental illness. In addressing the underlying chemical imbalances, we free the brain to heal, making new connections in response to positive stimuli. We also free the mind from the intrusion of perceptual disturbances, taking back the self once lost to trauma.

In cases such as Sylvia's, the complexity of her symptoms and pure breadth of reach required multiple management strategies. The thing to remember is that no patient will ever be the same as the one before and that medication that has faithfully worked for so many individuals may simply fail to show effectiveness in the patient before you. The key to psychiatry is no different than life itself. It is through a series of mistakes, guided only through trial and error, that one will discover the satisfaction of freedom from what ails them. You have to continue to motivate the patient for greatness. You have to be the voice in their head that gives them hope for a clearer tomorrow. Only then will they find the strength to stand up to their abuser and face the scars that lay below the surface.

CHAPTER 11

Psychosis

(THE RANTINGS OF A PSYCHIATRIST)

"When the mind betrays the self, we become teenagers in love with a woman who knows not of our existence. We dream of a woman's touch just as the brain dreams of a trusting mind."

When you hear the word *psychotic*, do you picture blood-thirsty cannibals? Do you picture some cliché horror film? The screams of a buxom blonde, as the psychotic killer slowly shuffles towards his victim. A stone-faced killer, fresh from his escape of the local insane asylum and now hell-bent on creating death and destruction? How about the example of an individual suffering from an untreated mental health disorder who shoots up his neighborhood or even a school, in a fit of psychotic rage?

Now that you've read some of the experiences I have faced as a psychiatrist, I hope that you have come to realize that these common depictions of psychosis, are that of outliers and their perception of being commonplace couldn't be further from the truth. Psychosis is nothing more than a symptom of a struggling brain and a mind trying to process information—a brain with irrelevant firings of synapses that could be induced by genetic predisposition, substance abuse, changes in hormonal and neurotransmitter concentrations, or any other of the numerous possibilities. Or maybe the brain is attempting to compensate for an overly sensitive nature to stress and stimuli, all while having limited resources to deal with the information currently bombarding the system. This combination results in a perception of truth that is skewed from reality. It is not a motivator of death and destruction and it is certainly not a definitive precursor for violence.

Psychosis is a general term used to depict the outward signs of individuals suffering from conditions indicative of misplaced reality. We may claim that reality is subjective, but in truth, human reality is considered absolute within agreeance of a population and resides as a state of all things as they actually exist. An existence free from idealism, perception, or subjective conditions.

Individuals with symptoms of psychosis may have delusions based in paranoia or grandiosity, while others may be tormented by perceptual disturbances in the form of auditory or visual hallucinations. Psychosis can also create functional impairments such as reductions in the formulation of linear thought and basic coherent speech, as well as limiting a sufferer's basic ability to comprehend information presented. An individual's thoughts, emotions, and behaviors may also be unusual, or even bizarre, while detached from the truth around them.

Most important to realize is that psychosis is a symptom, not an illness. Psychosis may last for only days or weeks; however, it can also linger for a lifetime, playing a part in a frightening, chronic condition. Such a prolonged condition may entail only subtle symptoms, while still allowing the individual to flourish. On the other hand, the condition could be more aggressive in impairment, causing inconsistencies in basic activities of daily living such as grooming, hygiene, and caring for oneself. With proper medication adherence, this same enduring condition could also present with complete remittance of symptoms with only occasional "flare-ups," or episodic reemergence of symptoms. These intermittent exacerbations are no more complex than that of simple emotional incontinence.

Psychosis appears to be likened to an unchoreographed routine of cerebral mismanagement coupled with a mind attempting to translate signals for which it is unfamiliar. This wake of foreign signals arises from deviations of connectivity. An unknown dialect within the constructs of traditional, linear, axonal language. The mind fuels ahead, trying to make sense of cerebral misfires in the presence of neurochemical fluctuations and other reasons for derivation from normalcy. The spectrum of disorders that revolve around and entail psychosis are extensive and at the same time more common than we care to accept.

What is psychosis? Psychosis is a description of mental derangement derived from the Greek word *psykhe-* (mind) and -osis (abnormal condition). Our society seems to have an overriding reflex to associate all psychosis with the well-known diagnosis of schizophrenia. This may be due to the common representations through media or simply due to the ease for which these pieces fit into such a diagnostic criterion.

Psychosis is a state of misperception of actuality, unique to each person, as the disorder for which they are afflicted. The first written account of the word "psychosis" is credited to German physician Karl Friedrich Canstatt in 1841. Canstatt used the term "psychosis" as an abbreviation of "psychic neurosis." At the time, the term "neurosis" referred to any disease of the nervous system. The coinage was introduced to better define symptoms of brain disease, distinguishing disorders that were thought to be disorders of the mind from those that were identified as "neurosis," which was thought to stem from disorders of the nervous system.

As previously conferred, psychosis is a symptom, or set of symptoms, such as hallucinations or delusions, secondary to a primary cause. Hallucinations are perceptual disturbances—perceptions of life's particulars that are actual deceitful betrayals of the senses. A hallucination is a sensation, or sensory perception, that a person experiences in the absence of relevant external stimuli. That is, a person experiences something that doesn't truly exist other than inside their own mind. A hallucination can occur in any sensory modality, be it visual, auditory, olfactory, gustatory, or even tactile. A hallucination is a condition of conviction that the presence of something, or someone, realistically nonexistent is subjectively authentic.

Auditory hallucinations are the most common of the hallucinations experienced in times of psychosis. These intrusions can have content of commentary describing a patient's every movement. Auditory hallucinations typically consist of one or more voices conversing, which may be comforting to the patient, or bothersome and intrusive. They can also be speaking to themselves or to the patient. When speaking to the patient, they can arise as derogatory, instructional, or command-type. Command-type is the most fear-provoking, as often patients will hear a human voice (or other entity) instructing them to do or complete certain acts. Some commands may be that of simple coercion, telling the patient to not take their medication, while other more ominous occurrences may instruct the patient to harm or kill themselves or others.

Perceptual disturbances in the form of visual hallucinations within a setting absent of substance abuse are direct brain pathology until proven otherwise. If you come to my office endorsing new-onset visual hallucinations, imaging of the head will be required with the initiation of psychopharmacological treatments. In fact, all new-onset hallucinations, albeit visual or auditory, require head imaging prior to an official psychiatric diagnosis. Visual and auditory hallucinations encompass a vast number of organic brain disorders requiring due diligence to explore the root cause. Hallucinations can be experienced in medical conditions such as temporal lobe epilepsy, delirium, dementia, focal brain lesions, neuroinfectious processes such as viral encephalitis, and cerebral tumors. This list does not even entail the vast overlap of conditions related to intoxication or withdrawal from substances such as alcohol, cocaine, amphetamines, and benzodiazepines.

Other designations of psychosis may be found in delusions. Delusions are simply false beliefs. However, these beliefs are often fixed and subsequentially very difficult to overcome even in the face of evidence to the contrary. Common delusions include the belief that someone is following, or monitoring, their behavior and conversations, usually due to some covert governmental agency. Another common delusion is that a person is suddenly blessed with extraordinary powers or abilities. Delusions may also be non-centralized, in the belief that people around them have abilities to influence their judgements and actions via reading their thoughts and inserting their own. Psychosis can also present with much more mundane symptoms including difficulties concentrating, completing tasks, or making decisions. Patients often express thoughts that are "jumbled" and may appear confused.

Hallucinations can often be meaningful to the person experiencing them. Many times, the voices are those of someone they know. Sometime these voices are derived status post-trauma, when the voices are that of the perpetrator, with content that is severely critical, vulgar, or abusive. Sometimes the voices have no relation and no connection other than that of being present for lack of logical explanation.

Maybe it's unfair to say hallucinations don't exist. *About one-quarter of the human brain is involved in visual processing, which is more than any other sense, yet* we are limited by particular wavelengths of the visual spectrum. It is often said that what we perceive, and what we subsequently base truth upon, is only 1%. We discern most of our reality based on visual processing, yet 99% of visual information is not available for our input. With our perceptions only containing a small percentage of true reality, to act as though the concept of reality is familiar is foolish. A great rift remains between what we recognize to be real and what we logically determine to be true.

On a neurological level, seeing is truly believing. Maybe what we should say is that, in the presence of psychosis, the perceptions of reality are incongruent with commonly accepted social norms. It is important to preserve respect for a person's subjective reality, and prior to initiation of antipsychotics, I routinely ask the patient if they want me to free them from their perceptual disturbances. To remove the voices, visual hallucinations, or delusions, barring the patient is not an imminent danger to self or others, should be entirely up to the patient. Some find comfort and freedom from loneliness in the voices that pursue them. Some people find auditory or visual hallucinations to be merely a component of their religious experience. Throughout time, in particular cultures, these alterations in perception provided a label to the affected person as someone who is especially close to their deity, or one that is chosen. However, in some cultures, these perceptual disturbances are perceived to be the works or influences of evil entities.

The causes of psychosis are many, encompassing countless medical and mental disorders, all unique yet often with overlapping symptoms. These symptoms often lead to a psychiatric misdiagnosis while the primary etiology of this frightening compilation of symptoms lies cunningly disguised in the shadows of physiological misinformation.

Schizophrenia is a mental illness that identifies itself with psychosis as its primary symptom; however, schizophrenia also leads to numerous other symptoms, often just as debilitating as the disintegration of subjective reality. Schizophrenia presents with such symptoms as disorganized speech and behavior, catatonia, and what are deemed "negative symptoms" such as avolition and diminished emotional expression. The caveat is that schizophrenia will always present with psychosis, yet symptoms of psychosis are not always indicative of a diagnosis of schizophrenia. When someone without a historical diagnosis of schizophrenia suffers from symptoms of psychosis, we consider this a psychotic episode with vast possible etiologies requiring in-depth analysis. The mental health professional must always look upon a psychiatric disorder as a diagnosis of exclusion, and only after all pathological processes have been ruled out.

Thought disturbances are also common in people suffering from some form of psychosis. Often, these disorders are apparent simply via a conversation, noting form and flow of language. Thought disorders have particular identifications such as tangentiality, as one example, which occurs when speech wanders off target, in a fashion that is both illogical and unfocused, never to regain correlation to the initial subject of discussion. A patient can also suffer from a symptom labeled as poverty of speech, which is defined as diminished total verbal output. Another similar symptom revolving around thought and execution of speech is known as poverty of thought, which is defined as verbal output that may be adequate yet containing no significance of meaning. Thought blocking is another very common example, and one which often presents when a patient is attempting to converse with someone in reality yet at the same time ignore the communication inside his own mind. This can be obvious during conversation due to its abrupt deviation of course to silence, all as the auditory intrusions disrupt focus and bombard the senses.

At times, some people with schizophrenia may appear inexpressive, withdrawn, or unmotivated. This is an element labeled as a negative symptom. This is often misperceived, or misdiagnosed, as a condition of major depressive disorder. These patients begin to isolate from their previously known existence, attempting to cope with this barrage of stimuli and paranoia. Often these individuals, still possessing insight of adequate understanding, begin to realize their previous life is crumbling before their eyes, adding even greater weight to an already complicated and grim circumstance. These negative symptoms can result in feelings of hopelessness, and often these mood alterations can lead to suicidality. It's important to note that patients with schizophrenia are at a greatly elevated risk of completed suicide.

Aside from a diagnosis of schizophrenia, there may also be a plethora of heritable characteristics, each increasing the likelihood that a particular person may experience psychosis. There is a hypothesis that individuals who are overly sensitive emotionally, and in temperament, may be more likely to experience psychosis if exposed to particular life events such as hardships, abuse, or trauma.

Another hypothesis is that of "epigenetic" influence, also known as the two-hit hypothesis. Let's use schizophrenia as an example. The theory in its most basic sense states that those who are genetically predisposed (hit #1) may be without disease if not encountered with a particular stressor. Those who are exposed to a particular life event (hit #2) may have activation of those genes for schizophrenia. This leads to downstream changes in specific proteins, leading to a cascade that ends with the production of schizophrenia. Basically, the gene is there, but its activation may depend on outside stimuli provided by their environment. That environment could be severe stress, suffering abuse as a child, or even the once-thought-to-be-innocuous use of cannabis as a teenager.

The dopamine hypothesis is another potential cause, and prediction, for onset of schizophrenia or other primary psychotic disorders. Evidence for such is simple. Cannabis and other drugs, such as stimulants, increase dopamine in the brain. These substances are known to cause psychosis, most likely secondary to the increase in this neurotransmitter. Further evidence is provided when patients with psychosis are given medications, known as antipsychotics, which often give relief or resolution to the psychotic features. The downstream effect of such medications is an overall decrease of dopamine in the brain; therefore, one can extrapolate that dopamine plays a role in psychosis. How do we know that antipsychotics decrease dopamine? Well, if you give a patient an antipsychotic, one adverse effect that is relatively common can be that of Parkinsonism. We know definitively that Parkinsonism is caused by reduction of dopamine in a particular part of the brain; therefore, the mechanism of action is implied via an antipsychotic's potential for adverse effects.

It is important to remember that the function of all neurotransmitters is to convey information. Dopamine, for example, is used in the pathway that communicates social threat or fear through perceptual cues, and of course reward, hence the addiction potential for many substances. Therefore, it would make sense to think that if found in excessive amounts, communication between particular regions of the brain may be more active, stimulating disturbances of perceptual cues and breaks from reality. Some studies have also attempted to explain schizophrenia in observed differences in brain structure in people with a known diagnosis of schizophrenia versus those without. Some patients with schizophrenia display alterations from "normal" controls in volume of grey matter and differences in activation in brain regions, and some may have differences in size as well as structure of the hippocampus and the amygdala.

As a species with a large and fortuitous cerebral cortex, we are constantly processing and interpreting the world around us. Like any higher-level functioning machine, the brain can, and often does, make mistakes. The brain is also subject to pure laziness simply filling in gaps of reality to take a shortcut. Sometimes the connections our brains make can be skewed or altogether flawed. Even with such shortcomings, humans have succeeded in many great accomplishments. With all our evolution comes a price, and those that succumb to such misfiring of the computer inside their head deserve our empathy, assistance, and respect.

Many questions arise when we start to explore more scientific roots of psychosis as found in schizophrenia, among many other mental disorders. We are abounded by theories that seem to fit in particular scenarios yet dissolve when positioned to answer alternatives.

Historically, theories on the origin of psychosis were much more straightforward. The inquest for explanation of such was to simply chalk up such symptoms as being related to demonic possessions or gifts from a supreme being, or even to haphazardly blame them on developmental psychological processes due in part to rejective or overprotective mothering.

In the 1930s, researchers set out to determine the cause of schizophrenia and found a willing population in the families of these patients eager for treatment and prayers for a cure. What the researchers determined was out of the 45 schizophrenic patients analyzed, over 75% had been subjected to what was designated as either maternal overprotection or maternal rejection. This led researchers to deduce that with the high prevalence of such similar maternal predispositions, this must be the insult that drives a normal child to psychosis, and the term "schizophrenogenic" mother was born. It was more or less a theory that normal children were driven mad at the hands of unstable mothers and the patterns of schizophrenia displayed by a child growing up was simply a way to cope with such an unforgiving environment. This theory held until its debunking in the 1970s after research displayed no higher prevalence of schizophrenia in children with such labeled schizophrenogenic mothers in comparison to mothers who were deemed psychiatrically sound. In hindsight, the theory of schizophrenogenic mothers seems a little embarrassing in its simplicity for such a complex disorder.

Our last common ancestor to the great apes emerged from its lineage 6 to 7 million years ago (using current estimates of divergence). Our ancestors did such with a path to future adaptations while developing the ability to walk upright. This bipedal ambulation was gifted through adaptation in spinal curvature, along with hip and lower extremity changes to support the body's weight. We also developed initial and persistent incremental changes allowing us to accurately throw objects due to structural adaptations in shoulder anatomy.

Most important of all evolutionary adaptations was the evolution in language, and with an increased nutrient-rich diet came accelerations in overall brain size. This size was not only in overall mass but also in available area leading to proliferations in neuronal connections. With this came higher cognitive functioning, all thanks to the folds of the neocortex, leading to further progression of thought and creativity. It is postulated by some that while our knuckle-dragging cousins continued to climb trees and find sustenance from a mostly fibrous and fruit-filled diet, our ancestors increased their caloric content of protein leading to linear growth in brain size. With this neocortex, and its substantial increases in complexity, came the potential for miscalculations between the brain and mind. Such miscalculations would eventually give way to perceptual disturbances in some members of the species; however, the age of onset was late enough to not affect procreation and subsequent genetic lineage being passed to future progeny.

To understand the implications of such higher brain functioning, we can explore the very limited witnessed accounts of psychosis in any animal species outside of Homo sapiens. Granted our attempt to discover examples of psychosis outside our species is limited, if not absent, our ability to study psychosis in humans is plentiful in its spectrum of subjects.

Schizophrenia is one mental illness that, while common in humans, appears to have been spared in all animals. Maybe schizophrenia will simply remain an unfortunate price we as humans pay for our large and overly complex neocortex. What gives us bipedal primates with opposable thumbs such capacity for language also may predispose our species to mental states of disarray. Maybe with the gift for complex calculations, self-cognition, art, and creativity comes the inherent risk of perceptual disturbances and emotional dysregulation.

Throughout history, the seriously mentally ill have often been viewed with distrust, aversion, and trepidation. During the Middle Ages, witchcraft and demonic possession were considered to be the root of emotional disturbances and confession, and exorcism found its place as a potential and plausible treatment. Many individuals with psychiatric disorders, as well as those with primary medical origins to their psychosis, including those with dementia, were tormented with spells, incantations, and rituals in order to oust what other-worldly forces possessed the unsuspecting victim. When witchcraft was later established as the cause of psychosis, individuals were tortured as a way of procuring a confession and to rid the subject from evil influences. Unfortunately, many such procedures peddled as a cure actually led to death.

The exploration of remedies for mental illness certainly did not stop there as further physical interventions were trialed. These interventions included bloodletting, either by the infliction of wounds or leeches, induction of vomiting to eliminate poisons, and the barbaric practice of trepanation, which involved the boring of holes into the skull with the misguided purpose of releasing evil elements from the mind. When all else failed to provide symptom remittance, the individuals were forced to succumb to a crude form of electric shock without anesthesia or paralytics. This electricity triggered seizures of such violent severity as to cause the patient to break their own back by the sheer force of the person's own clonic spasms and subsequent muscle contractions. When patients were found to have psychosis refractory to previous attempts, and if they had survived such procedures, then they were left to face physician-assisted insulin shock, or to face the permanence of frontal lobotomy.

Thankfully, the discovery of the antipsychotic chlorpromazine in the early 1950s launched the era of modern psychopharmacology. What would become an ever-growing class of medications displayed efficacy in alleviating some of the most disturbing positive symptoms of the psychotic patient, helping to initiate the unearthing of the neurobiological processes underlying these disorders. These medications helped usher in a new era of treatments and to the dissolution of the cruel and inhumane treatments of the past.

Maybe the most important connection is not the history of such disease states, their causes, or their cures, but the way in which we approach fellow humans suffering from such diseases, mental or otherwise. The most life-changing aspect of care is not a complete understanding of the disease, nor the medications used to treat such. Instead, it is the organic and empathetic connection we make with sufferers of mental illness.

When treating the mentally ill, it's important to show patients humanity and to be present with an open and honest mind during interactions. I tell them when I am confused or unsure of a disease course. I tell them when I have no idea when they will get better or if a particular medication will work for them. However, I always present the patient with comforting positive outlooks. I let them know that we are a team, and as a team, we will find the answer together. I explain to my patients that this is not a one-time-and-done type of situation, it's a relationship. In this relationship, we will work together to find what works for them. We may learn what ten drugs don't work before we find the one that does, but when we do sift carefully through that pay dirt and come up with a big golden payday, it will all be worth it.

CHAPTER 12

Custody of Self

CLARA

"What a wonderful day for an exorcism!"
—The Exorcist (1973)

The only things that scare me are those that I cannot control. I avoid feelings of helplessness at all cost. I cannot fathom the horrific sensation of an unholy entity—call it a spirit, ghost, or demon—seizing control of the body, consuming the sense of self, and discarding free will. While this possession of form is controlled like a puppeteer via a ventriloquist, the brain comprehends the infestation, but the mind, powerless to overcome such an intruder, struggles to break free. Unsuccessful, one is forced to watch their body disintegrate internally from the evil within.

On day 3,722, I meet with Clara, a 32-year-old Hispanic female, who initially came to me for treatment of her first episode of psychosis. Her disorder, which came on abruptly, was status post a very painful divorce. The former husband had decided on a new bride and did everything he could to destroy every part of Clara that remained standing. He obviously took the vow and sanctity of marriage to be construed as temporary until a greener pasture presented itself. Instead of a lifetime longing to remain in love, he destroyed all that was his former life. With threats of having her deported or worse, he basically blackmailed her into signing away custody of their children and any financial support. This left her homeless, broke, and unable to care for herself. She was forced to live with her sister and brother-in-law who were kind enough to open their home.

After our first meeting and after hearing her story, I am taken back at the aggression and callousness her former lover had perpetrated—all these stabs to a woman who already stood bleeding from divorce. According to her, they were happy until he became tired of her and his gaze fell upon another. I decide right then and there that I will not let her down as so many other men in her life had done up until this point.

"I'm going to see you every week until you get better! Okay? I am going to be here for you until you get your life back on track. We are going to work on the voices until they disappear. Then we are going to work on getting you a job you enjoy, your own place, and then, most importantly, regaining custody of your children. Does that sound like a plan?"

She begins to sob and simply nods her head to indicate yes. Her emotion is so raw yet in a sense relieving, as if the tears were an indication that all hope is not lost. Can I assure her the voices will go away, she will get a job, and she will eventually get her children back? Of course not, but I can sure as hell try. Sometimes all people need is positivity, support, and a little medication. Such a simple recipe can change lives and open doors once thought to be permanently closed.

I see her every week for the first eight weeks until nearly all her symptoms of psychosis were in remission. At that point of stability, we begin to decrease the frequency of our visits to every other week, and eventually, as things progress, once a month.

I watch amazed, as at this point her strength is what drives progress and I serve the purpose of being nothing more than a spectator. One would be at odds to recognize the woman before me as the same who presented less than six months previous. The woman who originally appeared beaten and defeated had risen to something unrecognizable. Even the tone of her voice now commanded respect. Her current success makes me doubt my original preconceived notion that she was a woman emotionally and physically broken as now I realize her bruised exterior did little to reflect her intact ambition and determination. The temporary scars of blue and black hues for which she initially presented meant little to the formidable presence and power she held underlying in reserve.

Over those seven months, she was not only able to surmount an effective defense to the auditory hallucinations but was also able to find employment at a major department store, and in true nature of success, had a job she actually enjoyed. She saved and was able to procure her own place, and with a little help from a pro-bono custody lawyer, she is awarded full custody of her three children. How such a great lawyer just happened to call her, out of the blue, to represent her for free is still a mystery. I guess some mysteries are left better unsolved, wink, wink.

Over time we are even able to titrate down on her antipsychotic medication of aripiprazole, and she continued to function well at a much lower maintenance dose.

From this vantage point, all is well with the world and things continue to go well, up until that point where they don't. I find myself surprised when I see her on my schedule a mere two weeks after one of our previous meetings, especially since we are on a four-week timetable at this point.

I quickly get up from my desk and poke my head out of the office. Here, I verify the appointment with my secretary, who assures me this is not a mistake. Apparently, she called in early this morning requesting an emergency appointment with me. I back up into my office and pause. I go over the last appointment in my head, failing to recall any red flags, social changes, or medication changes. I would be lying if I said I wasn't concerned; however, until that appointment, I have other patients that require my full attention. I simply bury my mind in work until she arrives.

When her appointment time comes, I hurriedly go out into the waiting room, not lingering in my office for the secretary to facilitate the patient encounter as I usually do. I find her sitting in the waiting room with her brother-in-law. Cautious not to alarm them with my own concern, I give them my safest wave and usher them into my office.

As normal, Clara presents well. I simply let her talk and tell me about all the recent stressors in her life, none of which are rather worrisome. I begin to get the impression this visit didn't require the anxiety I previously granted it. I begin to steer the course of conversation toward the reason for the emergency appointment.

Just as she attempts to tell me about her most recent derailment from stability, her body begins to shake. This shaking progresses to a series of wild gyrations, until her head is thrown backward, and her spine is curled over the back of the chair. At this moment, her mouth, already wide open, begins to expel a drawn-out growl that is quite unnerving. It is at this point that whatever, or whomever, has garnered control of this young woman's body speaks.

"We will not let you talk to her!" Her voice, while extremely deep, still has a human quality.

In this moment of utter shock, all I can muster, after all my years of study, is, "What the hell?"

I stand up from my chair and step quickly around my desk towards her. Her face is seemingly being stretched by all the muscles in her head. Her eyes are wide open. Her mouth is spewing a rumble of demonic possession, reminding me of the low-pitch growl synonymous with the movie *The Grudge*. If pressed, I would describe it as an unpleasant, metallic, death rattle of a sound. Obviously, that is not the most accurate descriptive term and not to be confused with the clinical occurrence of the "death rattle." That is the sound someone produces when near death, as the saliva and bronchial secretions begin to pool in the patient's throat and upper chest. This is clinically known as terminal respiratory secretions or simply terminal secretions, also known as the "death rattle."

I stand part doctor concerned for her safety, waiting for a chance to assist, and part scared Christian. I hope my statement of, "What the hell," is merely an expression and not that of an explanation.

Please don't let it be an explanation, I think to myself, for if this entity was to detach from its current victim, I would be in range for secondary possession. I wonder to myself, *Is secondary possession even a real thing?*

I attempt to extinguish my internal dialogue, all the while wishing I had brought a wooden cross and holy water to work today. I should have been better prepared.

The episode I am witnessing is over within seconds. Upon its cessation, Clara continues, completely unfazed, picking up from the previous sentence that was interrupted. As she continues to talk and act as if nothing happened, I find myself perplexed by the lack of discussion regarding the elephant in the room.

"Wait, wait, wait! Clara, what the heck just happened?" I ask.

Without hesitation, she answers, "It was the voice inside me, talking through me."

"Whose voice is it?" I again struggle, stumbling for clarity.

She replies rather calmly, "It's someone else's voice. I don't know who, though. It just takes over my body."

"When this other voice takes over, are you aware? Are you aware of what the voice is stating?"

"I am aware when it happens and most of what it is saying, but I can't do anything about it."

Similar episodes occur with unnerving frequency during our 50-minute assessment. Each episode, regardless of duration, is followed by an instant state of clarity, with her continuing the previous conversation as if the short interval of possession never occurred. She never appears to be in pain, nor does she lose consciousness. She doesn't seem to suffer from post-ictal confusion and appears relatively well, when not in this dissociative state. I think that this must be some type of rare seizure activity, while also realizing, with a high probability, that I may be wrong.

I do not claim to be a neurologist by any stretch; however, 20-30% of psychiatric residency training involves training in the field of neurology. It is an important educational aspect in the diagnosis of psychiatric disorders and an essential tool to distinguish ailments with a neurological origin versus those of non-related, psychiatric derivation. To give further examples involving neurology's role in psychiatry, one only needs to look at the national governing body for psychiatry. It is referred to as the ABPN, or the American Board of Psychiatry and Neurology. This organization also proctors the psychiatric board exam, which all psychiatrists hoping to become board certified must successfully pass. In this exam, a large proportion of questions will also relate to neurological conditions and complications arising from such. This is done to assure all board-certified psychiatrists are competent and comfortable with neurological diagnosis and organic rule outs in the face of psychiatric symptoms.

With Clara's consent, her brother-in-law chimes in frequently during our assessment, giving detailed accounts of these worrisome episodes. He confirms its initiation without preceding warnings and states the episodes continue without cessation. He confirms the absence of drug use or witnessed antecedent traumatic head injuries in the weeks and months prior to Clara's decompensation. He also endorses occurrences witnessed during times in which Clara has no knowledge she is being observed. This will help appease those suggesting states of non-epileptic seizures, also referred to as "pseudoseizures," and help exclude theories of a purposeful or factitious presentation.

I ask Clara, and her brother, to present to the emergency department after our assessment for a CT scan and neurology consult. With her already on an antipsychotic, I add a mood stabilizer, which has the secondary mechanism of being an anti-convulsant. Feeling this may be seizure activity, I cannot in good conscience let this woman leave my office without medications for potential seizures, especially in the face of concurrent antipsychotic medication use, which alone has been proven to lower the seizure threshold. I know damn well that a neurology consult in the setting of the emergency department is most likely not going to happen in the absence of stroke criteria. Clara will be forced to make an appointment with her primary care provider. This provider will then prepare a referral to the neurologist. This entire merry-go-round of doctor visits could take weeks to months, all prior to an actual human-to-human appointment. That is much too long a wait for an impatient, and unfortunately somewhat impulsive, personality type such as mine. Not to mention I could not bear to know one of my patients is suffering because I chose to wait for a neurology consult rather than rely on my training. Many physicians choose to stay strictly within their scope of practice to lower risk of being sued should potential problems arise. This is a common technique known as C.Y.A., a.k.a. *Cover Your Ass.* This is not to say I'm willing to perform cholecystectomies or breast augmentations; however, in my opinion, medications related to the field of neurology are certainly within my capacity, hence this initiation of medication for possible seizure activity in an outpatient setting.

I stand up and walk them both to the door. I repeat the plan once again for good measure, overviewing the medications and side effects for a second time. As soon as Clara reaches the hallway, she turns, thanks me, and continues to initiate her travel down the long stretch of white walls toward the exit. As she moves forward, she stops only ten feet into her journey. Her entire body begins to writhe in rhythmic fashion. Her brother-in-law attempts to hold her upright, but her body's jarring is much too intense for his grip and she falls to the ground. No sooner than her backside touches the ground does her back again arch, allowing her head the opportunity to slowly lower to the ground. All this transpires with the prior unpleasant soundtrack from hell, expressed from somewhere inside her. After what seems like minutes, her eyes fixate on mine as I kneel next to her. She slowly rolls towards me in an attempt to rise from the floor, but I gently place my left hand on her right shoulder, instructing her in a calm voice, "Just rest. Relax, Clara." I leave my hand on her shoulder to provide comfort as well as to maintain her position on the floor.

I ask the nurse to call for EMS while I continue to monitor Clara. Someone hands me a jacket, which I'm guessing is their attempt at treatment of possible shock. I thank them, take the jacket, roll it up, and use it as a pillow for her head. I see the displeasure in the jacket-provider, but I couldn't care less at this moment. My only concern is that for the safety and comfort of Clara. While waiting for the cavalry, we perform the most basic of functions, such as a finger stick for blood sugar, pulse oximetry, and basic neurological testing.

EMS arrives shortly, and after a quick update regarding Clara's disposition, she is transported to the local emergency room. I take proper action and call ahead to speak to one of the doctors in triage. This is typically done to provide valuable information as well as to expedite my patient's treatment. There is an unspoken agreement between outpatient doctors and their emergency room counterparts, that if we communicate via phone prior to a patient's arrival, that patient will be quickly funneled through the vetting process of triage.

Approximately two hours after the time Clara is placed into the ambulance, I receive a follow-up call. The call is from the same physician I spoke to earlier, giving me a courtesy update. He tells me that the CT scan of the head showed a large arachnoid cyst at the location of the cerebellopontine angle. Since arachnoid cysts in this region are rare, an MRI was performed to confirm the CT findings. The hospitalist in charge of admissions determined this was benign, not the cause of presenting symptoms, and was planning for discharge with outpatient follow-up. I abruptly cut him off and reiterate that this patient *must* be admitted for evaluation with an EEG (electroencephalogram) for seizure activity as well as for observation secondary to acute neurological changes. Oddly enough, the request of a resident physician is granted, and Clara is admitted. A small win for stubborn resident physicians everywhere.

What transpires over the next 24 hours is a shitstorm of attempts from hospital staff to get this "psych" patient out of the hospital. If over that day, I had a dollar for every time I heard the pathetic excuse for a punt, "It's just a psych issue," I'd be able to take myself to Chipotle for lunch every day the following week.

What is a punt? Well, the act of punting is a term used in football (American football). It is used when a team has used up all of the attempts to score and now just says, "Fuck it. Kick it to the other team and let them play with the ball for a bit!" In medicine, it's pretty much the same thing. If you can't figure it out immediately, just kick the patient somewhere else. Making the patient someone else's problem is easier for physicians who don't like puzzles they can't immediately solve.

Unfortunately, not all puzzles are comprised of a simple twenty-piece cat portrait. Some puzzles are of a field of flowers with hundreds of similar pieces, each only slightly deviating from the next. It takes more than just patience to complete such a project. It also takes devotion to your craft and passionate determination to heal those in need. It takes time and energy to work up a case as challenging as that field of flowers. Unfortunately, in our current age of overworked medical practitioners, if you find yourself to be that patient with a puzzle comprised of intricate complications, get ready to feel the wind in your hair, because your ass is about to get punted.

The problem with the medical field is that psychiatric patients, those labeled as having a primary diagnosis of a mental disorder, will often become victim to assumptions that all future and often-unrelated symptoms have arisen secondary to that psychiatric diagnosis. I have seen psychiatric patients with chest pain that are turned away as just having anxiety. I have even seen a psychiatric patient in the midst of a stroke being mislabeled as suffering, not from a cerebral vascular incident, but from a panic attack all because he had the common antidepressant, Zoloft, on his list of home medications. This predetermined assumption failed amendment even as this patient presented with severe left-sided weakness and slurred speech. In regard to this particular incident, I was assigned to his case the following day, and upon initial assessment, I became immediately concerned and ordered a stat CT scan of this patient's brain. In my mind, I assumed the worse, yet affixed my best poker face as I spoke to his loving wife, who had been cemented to his bedside since admission. I prayed my own assumptions would be unfounded. It is a strange occurrence when you find yourself hoping that your training has misguided you and that what you expect is only a misled conviction created by that of an inexperienced resident physician. The results of the CT scan were quickly returned and with it the overwhelming realization that we had failed this patient. Although I had no part in his misdiagnosis, I couldn't help but feel guilty for what had transpired. The results confirmed that a recent and major stroke had caused an extensive area of ischemic brain damage. With the acute stroke treatment window having passed nearly 18 hours prior, this patient, and his family, would be forced to contend with the sequelae following the acute damage and the residual hardships likely to follow.

Curious as to Clara's progress, I head up to the third floor on Saturday, even though I'm not even on shift or call. As I push open the door to the north entrance, I'm immediately greeted by a flurry of nurses in disarray for the possessed patient I have admitted to their floor. Not far behind is the hospitalist in charge of her care who of course greets me with the standard, "Why is she here? She is not having seizures; these are psych issues." Just as I'm fielding this statement, another group of nurses approaches. They inform me that the patient was in a catatonic state overnight. Apparently, she made her way out of the room and was found slowly walking down the halls in an obvious attempt to elope from the hospital, even further tying together their encouragement for mental illness. Throughout the reports, I also learn that she suffered multiple episodes overnight, similar to those previously witnessed in the office. Obvious fear and confusion rest on the faces of those in attendance as, with much perplexity, they all try to remove the unnerving presence of this patient from their sight.

It is my job to see psychiatric illness as a diagnosis of exclusion. It is the physician's job—and yes, psychiatrists are physicians first and specialists in psychiatry second—to first rule out all potential pathological causes of psychiatric symptoms. The unique pathologies are numerous, and each has its own symptoms that mimic those symptoms indicative of psychiatric disorders. Much deliberation should be completed before branding a patient with a mental disorder. The diagnosis of a mental disorder is not one that I take lightly as I know the label will follow the patient for the rest of his or her life. All too often, people see this label as a definition of the self, complete with known societal imperfections. Patients go from humans enduring suffering to simply having a name tag that reads, "Psychiatric Patient."

I find Clara resting in bed. This previously healthy woman is now a product of bodily contortions and lip-smacking. When asked if there is any pre-seizure warning, which is called an aura, she recalls feeling her vision become "fuzzy" with a sense of being slightly off balance. She also reports seeing flashing colors just before she falls into one of her states.

As I personally peruse the head imaging that Clara was granted, I see the large cyst at the previously expressed location of the cerebellopontine angle. The cerebellopontine angle (CPA) (Latin: angulus cerebellopontine) is located between the cerebellum and the pons. The cerebellopontine angle is the site containing cerebrospinal fluid, meninges, cranial nerves, and associated vessels. Symptoms typically do not arise until the cyst has enlarged enough to cause pressure on the surrounding areas, also known as mass effect. Even when symptoms are present there is no guarantee of an accurate diagnosis, as these types of cysts often present with only discrete symptoms. With that being said, more symptomatic patients may be candidates for surgery. However, most lesions are treated conservatively with follow-up imaging to monitor for changes in size and disbursement, as cysts can increase in size causing symptoms to appear, especially if they press against a cranial nerve, the brain, or the spinal cord.

Arachnoid cysts are collections of cerebrospinal fluid contained between layers of arachnoid membrane that are present from birth (congenital) or may develop from head trauma. They are found in all age groups and account for about 1% of intracranial mass lesions. Very few patients will be symptomatic, and often these cysts are incidental findings on imaging. For the unlucky few with symptoms, they may experience headaches, seizures, impaired coordination of balance known as ataxia, dizziness, visual changes, and nausea.

Fortunately, no accumulation of cerebrospinal fluid is found in Clara's case, and no shifts or evidence of mass effect have been visualized. Unfortunately, without positive imaging indicating a seizure source and with only an inconclusive EEG, it's difficult to make any neurologist or hospitalist see potential for any cause other than that of psychiatric.

As one can imagine, Clara's time in the hospital is over before it starts. She finds herself discharged due to psychiatric complexity without a known source or medical origin. I see her the day after discharge in the outpatient clinic and take it upon myself to treat the patient's symptoms with the same mood stabilizer I was planning on initiating prior to her admission. I choose a medication called valproic acid, and within the first week, her number of episodes is cut in half. By the third week, she is completely free of suspected seizure-like activity, "psychiatric-induced episodes," or whatever the hell people want to label it as. Patient diagnoses are labels only intended to provide future medical professionals the most basic of information. Labels such as chronic liver disease, hypertension, and hyperlipidemia can be important when providing care for the unfamiliar patient. In stark contrast, a psychiatric diagnosis is much more complex, and when passed forward, they are often done so without context, symptom severity, and course of illness. With such limitations, the provider's interpretation is often based on his or her prejudice influenced by negative encounters with previous psychiatric patients. This can prove deleterious to the psychiatric patient seeking fair and appropriate medical attention. As for now, my only concern is the treatment of her brain-originating psychiatric abnormality and stabilizing Clara back to her previous baseline function. I give much less concern as to which box to fit her in.

At the time of writing this book, Clara is symptom-free and living a happy and healthy life with her three children in their new home—just the four of them taking on the world together. No exorcism needed.

CHAPTER 13

Jinn

HEATHER

"I have never seen battles quite as terrifyingly beautiful as the ones I fight when my mind splinters and races, to swallow me into my own madness, again."
—Nicole Lyons, Hush

Jinn are said to inhabit caves, deserted places, graveyards, and any surroundings consumed by darkness. They are said to be intelligent spirits of lower rank than that of angels and something altogether different from demons. According to some beliefs, Jinn hold amazing strength and can hide among us, appearing in human and animal forms. Also, Jinn are said to have the capability to possess a living entity, seizing control over the unsuspecting host's vocal, mental, and physical exploitations.

Religion remains a powerful concept influencing mental health, and many different religions acknowledge the Jinn as real creatures that form a world other than that of mankind, capable of causing physical and mental harm to human beings through meddling and overt acts of possession.

My first encounter with such an entity is on day 3,783, when my patient, Heather, introduces me to the concept of such an entity. Heather suffers from a condition known as bipolar disorder with psychotic features. This means that not only does she have to battle severe mood dysregulation of manic episodes reciprocated by severe depression, but she is also forced to contend with intermittent psychosis during acute exacerbations of her primary psychiatric illness.

My monthly appointment with Heather begins as most have; however, on this occasion, the nurse assisting me was kind enough to lead her to my office after attaining vitals, saving me the arduous 20-foot trek down the hallway to invite her in. Unfortunately, I'm still working on the previous patient's note and attempting to properly submit the medication changes we had discussed. I invite Heather in and offer her a seat. I explain to her how happy I am to see her with the caveat that I just need one minute to finish up. She nods and provides a smile indicating this is of no great infringement and sits quietly in the blue plastic office chair.

Without warning, and in the absence of obvious inciting factor, she jumps up onto the chair. She has little concern for the sanctity of my office, nor does she respond to my invitation to remain seated; instead, she stands defiant on the cheap plastic chair, while pointing to the hallway and screaming for me to share the excitement of such a creature.

Speaking to herself, she begins to make her words available for us all. "Jinn! Oh, I usually only see them in trees. Holy shit." Then silence fills the air as I begin to rise from my chair to intervene in this balancing act.

"I'm going to slap you for telling him." Again, she is speaking to the air as if this Jinn is right before her, obviously conversing in a tongue not foreign to her own.

"Heather. Please be careful." I request as I help her down from this perch of discovery. "Come on, now. I don't want you to get hurt. Tell me, what did you see?"

"I saw a Jinn. Those slimy mother fuckers love to cause trouble."

I decide to go no further down this road of psychosis, instead trying to investigate the underlying pathology at work here. Most people think of the bipolar patient as someone who impulsively sells all their possessions overnight to buy a train ticket to North Dakota so that they can open a "can't lose" business opportunity of mass proportion—one involving pre-assembled tiki huts for the backyard-Polynesian art enthusiast, which they believe to be prevalent in large numbers in the great plains of North Dakota. These patients, having so much on the mind with massive numbers of ideas, begin to falter in linear thought and become disorganized and tangential. It is often overlooked that psychosis can also play a major role in such a disorder.

In my clinical experience, I would say at least half of the patients I have examined with bipolar disorder displayed psychotic features during cyclic times of mania or severe depression. The psychosis in bipolar disorder is not found alone, but instead in the context of, and secondary to, extreme shifts in mood. There is often a sense of congruence between a patient's mood and corresponding psychosis. This additional deviation from reality serves only to further limit appropriate reasoning and often prolongs the course of illness. Psychosis in this patient population can be disastrous, often leaving the patient paranoid against accepting treatment. In phases of depression, this psychosis can manifest into dangerous command-type auditory hallucinations with content of instructions to harm or kill themselves.

When a patient has an added qualifier, such as psychotic features, it is common to feel comfortable in our abilities to treat such due to the sheer amount of previous psychosis successfully treated. We often assume each class of symptom will present as consistent singularities amongst different individuals. This is natural as our brains search for patterns to increase future chance of success, and as our brains struggle to automatize our identifications and subsequent actions, it's difficult for the psychiatrist, or any physician, to see repeated symptoms consistently and to not somehow become desensitized to the slight variation in presentation. In some cases, however, one plus one does not equal two, and the primary diagnosis is drastically affected by the specifier attached. This creates a scenario where presentation, progression, and response to typical treatment may be surprisingly unique. It remains pivotal to proper care that we stay vigilant in searching through the subtleties.

As I continue my assessment of Heather, she overruns my questions, abruptly returning to describing her personal interactions with angels as well as the obvious government coverups. At this time, she is convinced that special forces soldiers are housed in her home using cloaking technology to remain undetected. She believes this to be the action of the government to protect her, and her alone, from those wishing her harm.

Again, she turns her head and provides threatening connotation to someone not visible to my limited wavelength of sight. "I'm going to slap you for opening your mouth! This is your last warning!"

This impulsivity and difficulty in redirection remain constant throughout this assessment, and at its conclusion, very little insight has been gained into potential inciting factors. I am left only with a suitcase of symptoms and pending clinical judgements guiding my course of care.

I have known Heather for quite some time, and I can safely say that she is a product, not only of genetic predisposition, but also of historically severe spousal abuse. For years she suffered physical, emotional, and sexual abuse by a man who at one time claimed to love her. The scars upon her face never let me forget the previous agony she endured, while her current state reminds me of the suffering her mind has sustained.

On my next meeting with Heather, after the Jinn incident, she has a whole new batch of delusions to share with me—not in place of the Jinn, but in addition. She again begins our conversation before I knew it had begun. "You know there are holes in heaven?"

"No, I didn't realize that, but good afternoon, Heather. How are we feeling today?"

"Well, I'd be a hell of a lot better if angels would stop falling out of heaven."

I'm reminded of that cheap pick-up line, where the man approaches the woman at a club or bar and asks, "Did it hurt?" "Did what hurt?" she replies, obviously confused how this man would have intimate knowledge of her somatic complaints, considering she doesn't know him. "Did it hurt when you fell from heaven? Because you look like an angel." The woman smiles, just before turning to her friends to engage in a group laugh and mockery of such a pathetic attempt at finding love.

Okay, I'll bite for a moment. The entertainment property of her stories is second to none. The simple act of engagement with Heather often provides a plethora of unique moments from a brain misaligned in function and a mind struggling for sanity. I don't find entertainment or amusement in psychosis, but it can provide intriguing understanding into the possibilities our mind has to create chaos. Even more, though, I enjoy watching the person before me, slowly over time, regain some semblance of reality and some portion of their former self.

Attempting to find some clarification regarding today's dilemma, I inquire, "So, what makes you think angels are falling from heaven?"

"Cause it's in the Bible. God allows Satan to release demons to test us. Demons are fallen angels from heaven."

"Okay, that makes sense. Have you been tempted lately to do something?" I realize I'm grasping at straws, trying to figure out the underlying topic of this conversation.

Not only does she not answer my questions, but she goes even deeper into the gorge of madness she has found herself trapped in. "I need fentanyl. Can you prescribe me fentanyl?" She asks this as if it was just a normal request I receive from patients.

"What do you need such a powerful opiate for?"

"Cause I have been up for a week and my body is inflamed from chemicals in the water. I need fentanyl cause it's an anti-inflammatory."

"How about you ask your primary care provider to write you a prescription for ibuprofen? It's a much safer anti-inflammatory."

After a moment of silence, she responds in favor of my suggestion. "Okay, I can do that."

"I'm curious as to how you know your body is inflamed." I realize as the words leave my mouth that I may regret my decision to continue engagement into her derangement from reality.

"Astral projections," she replies, shaking her head side to side quickly as she lowers her chin and gives me a wide-eyed glazed. Her look reminds me of something a pissed-off teenager would do if you asked them a question that they assume you should know. It's certainly plausible that the delusions are so well ingrained in her as to seem like nothing more than common knowledge. Maybe she believes in her delusions so intently that she assumes it is the same reality in which others find themselves a part of.

"I must be honest with you. I have no idea what you're talking about. Can you please explain what astral projections have to do with your inflammation?"

"Reptilian people meditate so they can transfer themselves through space and time and take over my body. They tell me to do things."

At this point, if I had a mirror, I would see myself looking perplexed and so intently lost as to appear foolish, and not just lower level "I misplaced my keys" foolish, but the upper echelon of ignorance in situational awareness. I feel likened to that man in a foreign country who is attempting to converse with the indigenous population. Of course, they don't speak English, but he continues nonetheless in his foreign tongue, repeating questions both more slowly and with increased volume, thinking this will somehow merge the disconnection of divergent languages.

It is here, however, in which I do notice something peculiar. I detect a common theme among some of my past patients for which I have interacted extensively. They too reported being plagued or visited by some sort of reptilian entities. Maybe there is more to this occurrence than can be simply explained away as perceptual disturbances. Maybe there is some correlation to the tails we once had and this intrusive idea of reptilian-like humanoids. It's possible this is simply what lingers after many thousands of years of suppression—a primitive memory that remains hungering for inclusion but left captive and incarcerated in the most ancient part of our brains.

I decide to be more direct and attempt to impart some quest for knowledge. "Is there a chance this could actually be auditory hallucinations created by your own mind rather than the influence of the reptilian people?"

"No, this is not mental. It's really happening. I have other people's souls inside of me."

This theory of her personal soul being displaced by those of others is actually quite common and could be a misinterpretation of a symptom known as thought insertion. Either that or this could be part of an elaborate defense mechanism. However, until proven otherwise, I will have to favor mental illness over astral projections.

It's possible her mind seeks understanding for the seemingly foreign voices inside. This gives us a way to rationalize our own actions by placing the responsibility at the feet of others. I can only imagine the anxiety produced by the belief that your body is being hijacked by other souls and using you as an organic train station hitching a ride to the next unsuspecting victim. Yet, this explanation is still seen as less chronic and less stigmatizing than the admission of having a mental illness.

"They are going to find me!"

"Who is going to find you?" I ask.

“The Jinn. They meddle in everything we do. They are fixated on me. They just won’t leave me the fuck alone.”

“Well, how about we send you someplace safe where they can’t hurt you.”

“Where is that?” she asks.

“How about the mental health hospital?” I suggest this with elevated inflection and a sympathetic nod.

I begin to address the matter of inpatient admission as there is no safe way for me to adjust medications to the level of appropriate titration in the outpatient setting. Also, I would be unable to provide the necessary guidance and safety measures her current state requires. These, however, can all be accomplished at the mental health hospital. As usual, my recommendation for 5150 comes with a great sense of guilt and the ever-present sigh of disdain from patients.

In the county I currently reside, we have no voluntary mental health hospital admissions; therefore, it lies solely on the psychiatrist to find reason for such a desecration of rights. I take this removal of basic human rights and freedoms very seriously, and I only use such an intervention when there are no viable alternatives. Although the process is involuntary on the part of the patient, I still find it important to have the patient agree or, at the very least, have a basic understanding of why I am holding them against their will. It’s a complicated and scary time for a brain already struggling and a mind on the brink of collapse. It’s best in these situations to show large amounts of empathetic understanding. It is also imperative to relay to the patient clear reasoning for the decision and help them understand that this is far from a punishment but in fact a gesture of caring, paternalistic medicine. What we don't want is to instill in the patient's mind that when they confide in a psychiatrist, they risk being punished with a vacation to a locked psychiatric ward.

Heather is admitted to the mental health hospital shortly after the cessation of our interview, and she is subsequently released ten days later. This is the last time that I will have to even contemplate the necessity of involving involuntary admission with Heather's course.

Over the passage of our time together, her mania remains persistent in its influence, but not with the previous severity. Her psychosis encased in her delusions persists, but perceptual disturbances gradually lessen with equal decline in intensity. Things progress as such until one day her brain appears at rest, coinciding with her mind. The generalized confusion between the two appears lifted and placed back into a shared reality. It is our sixteenth visit in eight months when a change begins to present itself.

Her presentation on this day appears no different than that of her sister who now accompanies her. She sits calmly in the chair across from me. No wild fluctuations in mood. No appearance of paranoia. Just sitting and present in the moment. For the first time, we share the same subjective reality, and for the first time, I get to truly explore her history. Her fulfilled dreams and lost hopes. The loves and pains of her life. The joy she experienced as a secretary for an accounting firm. I learn about her mother, whom she holds dear to her heart and would often quote in previous and future meetings. Heather's state of manic influence appears to have been resolved.

The road of bipolar disorder is that of a spectrum—a spectrum unique in experiences, and severity, amongst different individuals. Not uncommon along this spectrum are wild fluctuations found within the same individual. Despite my best efforts, Heather's mania lasted no less than six months, which for me was astounding. Typically, mood stability is garnered by medications in a much-shortened course. Some, however, are resistant to treatment and others are poor responders to the typical medications used to combat such an acute phase; even fewer patients, such as Heather, are both.

We continue to meet once a month, and over the last four months of my time at the rural outpatient clinic, I learn a great deal about Heather. I grow fond of her imagination as well as her strength through adversity. When she expresses ideas in a levelheaded manner, it becomes obvious that she possesses the gift of being quite influential, especially in regard to Jinn. Even in her baseline state, she has what some would consider problematic delusions. I tend to believe, however, that imagination and wonder are important for some humans who have trouble finding substance in life. Some people's lives are so very monotonous that intrigue is actually healthy for the mind, giving it purpose. For some, it's a lifelong search for Bigfoot, and for others, it is the constant interpretation of all things state-run to be that of a conspiracy. For Heather, it is the presence of Jinn.

She no longer expresses the visualization of such, nor the conversing with them, but she remains steadfast in her belief of their influence. This is what I was hoping for, actually. I don't want her to lose that unique view in which she sees the world. I never want to rid her of interpretations I feel are invalid. Her trip to the mental health hospital had nothing to do with unseen entities. It was simply a way to treat and resolve the dangers of mania while at the same time keeping her safe. These dangers include the lack of nutritional intake, the deprivation of sleep, the psychosis that interferes with daily living, and the impulsivity that can be utterly devastating.

Not all thoughts misaligned with social norms are delusional, nor considered that of paranoia. Some beliefs are products of imagination and some remain in the simple absence of a connection to the brain's previous experiences. Let's be honest, we all want to believe that the sound in the woods on our last camping trip was made by a glorious and elusive eight-foot ancient primate. It's much more rousing to the soul and exciting to the spirit than believing it to be nothing more than a pinecone relieved from its perch above only to strike the forest floor. To this day, I can't be certain there are not actual Jinn, entities bent on influence, trickery, and instigating ruckus among us humans. In fact, their presence would explain much of the adult life I have experienced, freeing my soul from guilt and failures. Whether Jinn are real or not, Heather was able to move past her mania and live her normal life, which is a win in my books.

CHAPTER 14

Internal Storage

JANET

"At the root of all addiction is pain."
—Unknown

On day 3,890, I receive a phone call from the ER attending physician, and he gives me the rundown on the latest psychiatric addition to his unit.

"Patient's name is Janet. She's a sixty-eight-year-old female presenting for right-sided headache of intense pain with prolonged duration of nearly one week. Patient has previous history of lung cancer, currently in remission. Patient appears to be paranoid and delusional and believes her ex-husband placed a spatula inside her vagina." A long pause interrupts his presentation. I can only guess he is attempting to process his last statement and is now regretting its inclusion in his report. He garners the courage to continue. "She states she has been hearing voices since the spatula was placed in her vagina."

He pauses, once again, leaving me wondering if his patient presentation is complete or if he simply found himself amiss amongst the insanity that has entered his sterile ER.

Just as I am about to interject, he continues, "Man, I don't know how the hell you deal with this patient population."

"Very cautiously," I respond.

He gives a short nervous laugh. "Yeah, I bet."

He continues to detail the presentation. "Patient also feels she is being followed by Satan-worshippers. Apparently, she feels targeted by these unknown persons and is in fear for her life. Patient believes current headache to be a product of her ex-husband who is using a new surgical machine that allows for invasive medical procedures, all without the patient's knowledge of such intervention."

I give a little final giggle to justify the ridiculousness he is obviously feeling and to ease his discomfort as I'm nearly certain he has never used the word spatula and vagina in the same sentence before.

When I finally arrive at my destination, I hurriedly make my way through the bustling hospital drama, and after a few quick waves and superficial greetings, I find the patient's room. I enter her room after a diminutive, non-enthusiastic knock, knowing this is going to be a shit-show of disorganized conversation.

As I pull the shade open and before I can present myself, my qualifications, and my intent, she takes the reigns. "I'm going to tell you something and I need your full attention," she insists.

"Of course," I reply as I begin to take stock in what I am dealing with.

Janet is a scantily clad woman who appears much younger than her stated age of 68. She sits across from me, seated on the other stool in the room. She does this rather than take position on the exam table that most patients are automatically drawn to do.

Her dress is provocative, as are her mannerisms. She provides me with prolonged eye contact and physical incentives that seem to be congruent with her ensemble. She confidently displays the residual products of breast augmentation surgery, which are rather easy to spot, even for the untrained eye, as ridiculously round and perky breasts in a 68-year-old female are relatively rare. Coupled with the obvious lip enhancements, this patient screams histrionic personality disorder. Fashioned with a low-cut blouse, she does her best to lean over as much as possible, hoping to distract me. I, in turn, do my best to thwart her proposals. I overexaggerate my stare to her eyes, combined with appropriate time staring in the distance as to paint a picture of a man listening intently while in deep contemplation.

Her hair displays residual pink highlights with the extended date of such affixment, apparent in the length of her native root color. Natural brown roots, with intermixed hints of grey, are now competing with the failing vibrancy of the hot pink tones. Her make-up is exaggerated and holds representatives from the entire color wheel. Her love of blue tones is wildly apparent on her canvas of skin. Her lips appear assaulted with bright-red lipstick—lipstick that looks as if it was put on during a jarring roller coaster ride, the outlines of her lips used only as a vague suggestion. Regardless, they remain puckered in enhancement of inflated features. I interrupt my gaze of scrutiny and evaluation and bring my attention back to the matter at hand.

She continues what seems to be an act of interrogation, questioning my knowledge regarding worshippers of the demons below. "Now, you are aware of the satanic worshipers and cults tormenting and terrorizing people all over the United States, right?"

"Honestly, I'm was not aware of that, but you have my full attention. Please tell me more."

"Well, this town is infested with them. I have been followed by my ex-husband, who is a Satan-worshipper. He is in a cult and they follow me and do things to harm me. He blackmails me into doing things."

I ask for more details, knowing very well I may regret asking for the roadmap to her 24-hour roadside café of delusions. "What types of things does he make you do?"

"Have sex with him. Then he lets his friends have sex with me. It's all without touching."

Yep, I regret it already, I think to myself. However, due to basic constraints of physiology, I'm curious to dig deeper. "So how exactly does that work?"

"It's like a virtual reality type of machine." She shakes her head, as if about to add to this description, but thoughts fail to produce sound.

I allow her silence to be an indication that it's time to move forward. "Wow. That sounds scary. So, when is the last time you saw your ex-husband?"

"Oh, it is. Very scary!"

I pause awaiting an answer to my question, but her disorganization is on a wavelength currently adrift from my own. I attempt to realign her focus by repeating myself. "So . . . when was the last time you actually saw your ex-husband?"

"I haven't seen him since our divorce in 1987, but he is still around. I can hear him talking, all the time. I had an extramarital affair during our marriage, so he is trying to get back at me by ruining my life and having other Satan-worshippers terrorize me. He has been doing this for over thirty years."

"That sounds horrible. I'm so very sorry. Have you contacted the police?"

"No! Well, not today, but yes, I have. I think I called them yesterday. Oh yes, I did, now I remember. I called them after I heard the mob of Satan-worshippers talking about me, just outside my window. As soon as I ended the phone call with the police, my ex-husband screamed through my air conditioner, 'You just signed your death warrant!' I called the police back immediately and told them this as well, and they put me in an ambulance and brought me here. I'm not crazy; I always tell the truth. Do you believe me?"

Ugh. She said it. The worst four words in psychiatry. Possibly one of the top ten worst phrases in the English language. I'd rank "Do you believe me?" as sixth, sandwiched between number five, "The baby is yours," and number seven, "It's probably just a rash."

"Well, you have given me a lot to think about and process. What I can say for certain is that I think it's obvious you're suffering, and I want to do whatever I can to help you."

"Can you do me a favor?" she asks.

"Sure. What can I do for you?" The truth to my response is somewhat limited, as I may do it if it's something small and not excessively time-consuming, but if it entails anything involving creams or lotions, I'm out.

"Can you call UCLA and see if any machines like the one I was describing has been stolen? You know, the virtual reality ones? Then, can you come back and tell me what you found?"

Rather than overtly lie, I give her my standard bullshit response. "I'll see what I can do." I know calling UCLA would only waste their precious time and would also make me look like a complete ass for buying into my patient's delusion. I also know that my response, while not a complete falsehood, is still nothing less than a lie. This conundrum is common in medicine. *First, do no harm* is not as simple as it sounds. Just the mere presentation of the truth can be an emotionally harmful act. In a patient with fixed delusions within a state of psychosis, the factor for complexity is elevated exponentially.

When it comes to delusions, I try not to confront the deviation from reality directly until I have built a trusting relationship with a patient. I don't go out of my way to endorse the belief that he or she is an undercover CIA agent or that my male patient is pregnant with a human fetus in his rectum (yes, that is a true story). However, outward and blatant confrontation of delusions in the early stages of rapport building can be detrimental to patient recovery and to overall emotional stability. We want our patients to not fear physicians for the impending scrutiny they will receive. Instead, we want a situation of trust and respect, creating a precedence that will encourage these individuals to present to future medical professionals should the next time their delusions or emotions run astray.

Once I'm done talking with Janet, I do my due diligence and run the necessary labs. My first goal is to rule out measurable evidence of biological pathology as reasoning behind such symptom presentation. I also send her for a head CT to rule out any grossly abnormal pathology, including that of potential metastasis. Imaging tests come back negative, but a strange value returns from the lab work: amphetamine positive.

With the obvious intracranial etiology ruled out, I explore the other possibilities for her decompensation. After a few short hours of stat labs and imaging, I again enter her room and apologize for the wait she has endured. I begin to lightly, and circumstantially, ask about drug use. This is a question I usually ask all my patients; however, in my gross oversight, I never thought I'd have to ask if this 68-year-old woman before me was currently using methamphetamines (meth). Yet, if I had, she would have opened up immediately, as it becomes clear she feels there is no misguidance or wrongdoing in her behavior. She sees her meth use as the better of two evils when faced with what she considers severe symptoms of attention deficit disorder (ADD). In all reality, the chemicals she is snorting regularly may very well be the sole cause of her delusions, or at the very least, exacerbating an untreated and underlying primary psychotic disorder.

Let us explore what happens when someone snorts methamphetamines. Snorting, also known as nasal insufflation, is the primary route for those looking to expedite drug metabolism, which leads to an instant and sustained rush of energy. The active drug in meth is ephedrine, or a form of such known as pseudoephedrine. This nasal decongestant is mixed with household chemicals such as acetone, rubbing alcohol, iodine, gas additives containing methanol, drain cleaner, lighter fluid, match tips, lye, paint thinner, rock salt, and our man of many trades, lithium (commonly sourced from batteries).

So why would someone ever snort such a deadly concoction? Immediate euphoria mixed with increased energy and alertness coupled with a decreased need for food, water, or sleep. The body basically goes into fight-or-flight mode and does so without the external stimulus of being chased down by a hungry grizzly bear protecting her cubs. The euphoria created by meth stems from the heavy surge of the neurochemical known as dopamine. Unfortunately, in excess, dopamine is also known to lead to psychosis and Janet is a woman who has been immersing her aging brain in a bathtub of this euphoric and psychotic-inducing substance.

When I ask her about her drug use, she appears perplexed but not quite as confused as she should be.

"I was looking over your labs and I noticed you're positive for amphetamines. Are you messing with any drugs?"

"No way! I only use a little meth for my ADD. It helps me get things done around the house like chores."

"Okay. I can understand being tired, but meth is very, very dangerous."

"Oh no. The guy I get it from is a very nice kid, so I know I'm getting the right stuff."

I take a moment and try to wrap my head around her muddled thought process, one that would allow meth to be prescribed by a street pharmacist for lethargy and that would make this use allowable and necessary.

"There are a lot of things that could be causing your feelings of being tired. I will look into those for you if you want."

"No, it's okay, I only use meth sometimes."

"I can appreciate that, but honestly, there is no 'safe' use of meth. How often are you using it?"

She appears to ponder, calculating her frequency of use. "Well, I only buy it from him twice a week, and I never do more than two lines in a day. Sometimes I will go two days without using it at all."

"What are you doing during the days that you're not using meth?"

"I sleep."

I begin to get frustrated internally as I can assume every hour awake is spent using meth, only discontinuing use when her body literally crashes from exhaustion and lack of caloric intake. After numerous days of intoxication, the body can respond no longer. With reserves empty, the body reaches exhaustion and sinks into a state of mandatory respite. As my frustration begins to bubble up nearer to the surface, I realize that this poor woman is suffering, and this drug use is not only the cause of her psychosis but also a direct effect of her psychosis. I cannot tell which came first, the psychosis or the drug-induced psychotic state. Unfortunately, without a clear and lengthy washout period, I cannot diagnose her with anything but substance-induced psychosis.

All too often, persons with mental illness use non-prescribed substances to escape from their own reality—a reality spurred by the very mind that imprisons them. All too often these patients will be looked upon, not as people who are suffering from mental illness, but simply as drug addicts with poor life choices.

It's at this time that I pause and again assess the situation. I check her mannerisms, witnessing her flagrant paranoia and her emaciated structure. She is obviously responding to internal stimuli and appears to be having a rather serious conversation with someone other than myself. There is no way this poor woman can care for herself properly in this state, which makes her current dress and make-up even more impressive. She seems to be suffering from an inability to cope with life, yet still able to facilitate proper function in previously learned behaviors such as dressing, make-up, and flirting. In her current state of paranoia and disability, I can wager no benefit from releasing her back into the wild without a full and thorough psychiatric evaluation and some much-needed stabilization. I know of only one place that she can quickly receive all this. Now it's time to let her in on my plan.

"Janet, let's talk about how we can get you feeling better."

"Oh, I'm fine, honey. If you could just prescribe me Adderall or Xanax for my ADD, I would be fine."

"I really don't think either of those medications are appropriate for you for numerous reasons, one being your current use of meth."

"Well, if you prescribe them for me, I wouldn't have to use meth."

I purposefully refuse to process such a statement, continuing along my train of thought. "Well, Janet, I'm worried about you. I think what's best is for you to come in and stay with us for a little bit at the mental health hospital."

"Oh. No, thank you."

"As much as I want to let you walk out of that door, I cannot in good conscience do so and still call myself a physician. You have a lot of things going on, and I want to help you get your life on track and find freedom from your ex."

She pauses as she realizes that once I utter the words, she will be guided to a 72-hour hold for her own safety. As if she knows that arguing would be futile, she does little to change my mind.

"Will they get me housing?" she asks.

"Well, there are social workers that will visit you and you guys can explore all the services the county has to offer."

"Can I come see you after I get out?"

"We can certainly try to get you an appointment with me, but for now, let's get you feeling safe, okay?"

"Will they give me Adderall and Xanax there?" Her addicted brain is bartering with the mind to make a deal.

"There are numerous other medications that may be helpful to you. You can explore those options with your inpatient doctor."

She quickly utters what sounds to be, "I'm allergic."

"Excuse me? Allergic to what?" I ask, confused but also simply trying to make an exit from this room without engaging in further negotiations.

"To psych meds."

"Which psychiatric medications are you allergic to?"

"All of them," she states.

"What about Adderall and Xanax?"

"I'm not allergic to those. Those are the only ones I can take."

I giggle softly to myself due to the absurdity of the exchange. "Okay, Janet, you will have to discuss that with the other doctors. I am sure they will do their best to help you. You take care now, okay?"

I turn to the door and walk through the threshold to safety—safety from the mind-numbing event I just experienced. I hear her voice continue to speak and I can make out only a phrase before my footsteps carry me from her range of sound. "Okay, I'll see you."

I think to myself, *Oh, I'm sure you certainly will*, knowing the grip meth holds on individuals and its prevalence in our county. I shake my head and laugh softly just to keep my mind strong and my emotions sheltered. I know that if I was to take in the gravity of the suffering I just witnessed, it would certainly ruin any chance for a tear-free day. There are no tears from your psychiatrist today, knowing if I maintain a tough exterior, I have a greater chance of mirroring such hardy, emotional regulation inside.

CHAPTER 15

Plurality of One

DEREK

"A nightmare has taken hold of my body.
Lunacy has dug its way inside my mind."
—Amanda Steele

It's day 3,947 and I find myself oddly contemplating the severity of something far from my own standard conscious thought. I did not envision during breakfast this morning that later in the day I would need to analyze agony on such a grand scale.

I stand here, envisioning the pain produced by moving a kitchen knife from its perfectly comfortable position in a drawer, only to reposition such a utensil abruptly into your own abdomen. The willingness to do such displays a motivation of intent difficult to conceive.

I can't help my wandering curiosity as I question if the pain is more severe if done slowly. Maybe a quick thrusting action is best to lessen the overall discomfort of the procedure, the feeling of sharp pain as you break the skin momentarily taking away your ability to voice such agony. You stand fixed in an emotional stalemate as the blade cuts and pierces its way through the bowels. Creating irreparable damage, the blade sinks further. The knife, built for such a task, remains devoted to its purpose as it faithfully releases the contents of your intestines into the surrounding abdomen. Transitioning from sharp to dull pain, the pressure fills every nerve and synapse. The blade reaches its threshold as your abdomen meets your own hand, the blade's fixed handle resting on your bloodied skin as the only mark of success. Once the blade finds a home, I wonder if retraction of such would only increase the discomfort.

Does one leave this metallic piercing inside? Is there some possible relief if removed? I imagine both options are equally difficult to distinguish, especially with the constant and fluctuating intensities of throbbing anguish overcoming your brain's ability to process the condition. Excruciating pain that increases with every breath is magnified in intensity with every filling and expiration of the lungs.

According to his mother, Derek was always a cheerful and energetic kid—that is, until just before his eighteenth birthday. At this time, a visible change gradually started to become apparent, and over the next two years, Derek would progressively transition from a smiling, socially involved teen to one with little emotional response. Her once outgoing boy had converted to an existence withdrawn from peers, secluded from family, and teeming with paranoia. Derek continued to isolate himself to a sanctuary of shelter realized only in his room.

In the beginning, this once carefree teen began to slowly disengage from social interactions. His parents witnessed fewer and fewer friends frequenting the home, as well as their son's ever-increasing isolation to his room. These are the seemingly trivial incidents usually referred to in historical reflection when speaking with parents regarding initial recognition of symptoms. Parents will often remark on the initial lack of worry at such behaviors believing such to be nothing more than a stage. That quintessential stage, representing the juncture in a teen's life where rebellion commences and propagation of frequent retreats to their room in favor of loud music and social media, over the uncool normality of familial interactions, becomes commonplace. Of course, in hindsight, the recipe of symptoms appears easily noticeable and frightful in culmination, yet at the time of occurrence, such symptoms are gradual and progressive, rarely inciting parental concern. Of course, any time a child begins to show changes in behavior, including that of changes in affect, patterns, and increased isolation, a thorough psychiatric and physical wellness check should be performed to rule out depression, substance use, bullying, or any number of ailments that will show vastly superior improvement if intervention is timely and sufficient.

Derek was seen out of his chambers only for meals or to conduct frequent lower home inspections. Each journey to inspection would be met with caring words and affection from his mother, which only seemed to further segregate his old self from this new psyche. He became engulfed in mistrust of all, including his mother, often scuttling back to his underground war room for further planning. Derek's paranoia became an obsession, and his compulsion for relief was that of checking the locking mechanisms of all doors and windows on the lower floor of their two-story residential home. It became a game of cat and mouse as his mother would take refuge in secrecy and stealth, hoping to catch sight of Derek's actions. She remained steadfast, hoping with blind persistence that this would provide insight into an issue she could resolve.

As the isolation increased, so did Derek's ideas of paranoia, his silhouette often found persistently peering out the closed window blinds. Careful to only disturb one rung at a time, he would slowly raise and insert his eye into the newly formed gateway to the outside. Here he would assess cars and people, scrutinize movements, look for patterns and deviations of such patterns, all the while becoming increasingly concerned with the possibility of malevolent behaviors on the part of neighbors, postal employees, and anyone who happened to drive by. He would keep journals of license plate numbers and paste check marks next to each in reference to arrivals and departures.

His mother didn't seem to worry—at least not to the point of interjection—until he began to noticeably lose weight. He became so paranoid that he would no longer eat food that he did not witness being unsealed and opened. Water had to be in bottles and opened only by himself due to fear of potential poisonings.

The family's primary care provider ruled out bacterial and viral etiologies, obvious health issues via extensive blood workups, and even a primary eating disorder. The primary care provider did, however, correctly suggest Derek's mother seek out a psychiatric consult, and she wasted no time in making an appointment. Unfortunately, it was nearing the holidays, and due to a limited availability of outpatient psychiatrists, Derek was given an appointment twelve weeks away. Derek would not make that appointment, and the holiday season would give more anguish than merriment.

It was late October, and Derek was nineteen years of age and still living at home. He became more of a home decoration than the college-bound, star pupil for which he was destined. Conversations would emanate from his room, yet no one could be heard answering or responding. His mother would quietly creep down the hallway, hoping to gain some insight into his disposition, only to capture a one-sided dialogue between Derek and an unknown voice absent to those outside of his head. Occasionally, when these spoken words become that of agitation, she would quickly knock on his door. This was more indicative of someone "rolling through a stop sign" than an intentional warning of impending interruption. Throwing the door open she would often hope to find that he had snuck someone in the house. Finding him with a girlfriend or even a homeless person would be a relief to her at this point.

"I didn't care who was in there," exclaims Derek's mother. "I just wanted there to be someone, a real person that he was talking to. It would have been so much easier to accept and understand."

Her eyes begin to fill and leak a watery form of despondent grief. This fluid, created by a tortured and confused mother, proceeds to roll down her cheeks and into her mouth, prompting her to wipe such an intrusion with the back of her hand.

"Sometimes I wish all this was just from drugs and not something in his mind. I know that is horrible to say, but then we could get him help and the problem would go away. I have read that schizophrenia is forever, and I'm worried he has that. Do you think he has that? Do you think he has schizophrenia?"

I find myself using a partial lie of compassion. "Well, it's still too early to tell. There is a multitude of explanations for what he is suffering from. Let's take our time and not jump to conclusions." I call this a lie of compassion, as I know damn well that this is the beginning of schizophrenia, and it's actually difficult to even say "beginning," as Derek has been suffering from such symptoms for quite some time. I just don't have the energy to further dismantle the limited hope of an already distraught mother. Also, there is a slim chance that his suffering is something completely foreign to mental illness and there may be another physiological process at work. I cling to this strand of hope in justification of the misinformation I just verbalized to her.

I again attempt to assess the validity of my initial diagnosis and recall the details of the incident as provided to me by his family. On the evening of the incident, Derek's one-sided dispute was exceptionally hostile. It had escalated to the point that he was receiving obvious commands to do something vile. The inner derogatory content could not be heard but was easily conferred by his outward denials. Such an episode forced his mother to coax him out of this dungeon of sorts. She would lead Derek down the stairs to watch a holiday movie with the family. She so desperately wished to live in the portrayal of normalcy, even if they had to fake it.

As a parent myself, I can attest to the joy such normal situations produce. Something as simple as eating dinner with your child, at an actual table with chairs, can create a sense of fulfillment and accomplishment only found through the feeling of being a good-enough parent. Along these same lines, the simple beauty of watching a movie with your child, no cell phones or video games, just the family immersed together in a journey of wonderment and suspense, is something that brings great joy to any parent. He or she will ever so often step out of the immersion just to gaze at their child's eyes and facial expression, appreciating the excitement and suspense they are experiencing. Who ever knew observing another human as they watch a movie could be so satisfying?

On this evening, Derek, his mother, and his younger brother crowded together on the three-cushioned couch, all bundled under blankets trying to engage in a fictional tale of horror and distract themselves from the tangible terrors of their own reality. With wide eyes and stifled motivation to move, they all watched a mute serial killer dispose of characters one by one in a slasher film aptly named after the holiday in which it takes place. Derek had always been a fan of scary movies. Many of us also find an awkward sense of pleasure and a rush of excitement from being surprised or scared. It is an innocence of relief that keeps the attention rather than some seemingly dark, macaw idealism.

As the movie progressed, each family member found themselves enveloped in their own survival. No one noticed Derek get up and walk out of the room until he had returned standing behind the couch with a movie-inspired hockey mask covering his face. When his mother called his name, Derek simply stood motionless. His mother took stock of the situation as she saw a large kitchen knife catching the flickering light of the television. She watched, in great agony, as Derek slowly raised the knife into view. She remained frozen in shock, unable to utter a word as horror gripped the moment. Astute only in shock, she was unable to formulate a method of intervention before Derek sank the knife just left from his midline, into his stomach, and just below the diaphragm. Both mother and brother sprang from the couch, screaming through their ascent. Not knowing if it was safe to approach, they remained across the couch, which seemed to create a suitable barrier of pleather and foam. It wasn't until Derek fell to his knees and limply to his back that they had the opportunity to approach. Derek's mother recalls moving towards and kneeling down next to her son to assess vitals, only to find Derek unresponsive. At the same time, Derek's brother called 911, doing his best to detail the happenings to the emergency operator. With the phone still to his ear, Derek's brother kneeled down behind his mother, resting his head on her back as he began to sob.

When I first meet Derek, it is five days after this incident. Fortunately, he missed all major organs and was stabilized rather quickly. At first sight, I see a young and rather thin man lying in a hospital bed amongst a team of worried physicians and staff. The crowd of onlookers is not so worried about Derek as a person, but rather as a liability. A severe suicide attempt, like the one he participated in, is a nightmare for practitioners. They remain enveloped in fear regarding the liability should they prematurely release him home, realizing a possible civil suit should he make another attempt on his life. They picture themselves in court trying to explain to a judge and jury their reasoning for discharge. It's enough to make the most seasoned physician question his capacity to make educated decisions. Though we can never know for certain if or when an individual may attempt to end his or her life, we do know that a psychiatric consult is great at saving the ass of the primary team so that all future attempts of suicide, and civil liability for such, now lie on the psychiatric team.

Fortunately, I do not share that same measure of concern, as a courtroom scares me little in comparison to the loss of a patient for whom I have cared for. I have lost patients to suicide, and when it has occurred, there is no greater sense of helplessness. I have spent days alone, canceling all other appointments, engulfed in tears, all while wondering what happened after their course and where it all went wrong. My only solace is knowing they left my hands hopeful and motivated for life. I blame reality and its cruelty to those who are trying to piece together a life with limited support. Even with these losses, I refuse to practice scared medicine. I do my best, with the best intentions, and realize I do not command any say over the world or the children within it.

Derek is a rather simple consult, as part of my current rotation is to determine the necessity for a 5150 hold and facilitating placement at a mental health hospital for stabilization. This is an easy choice for me as I have one simple rule: if you shish kabob yourself with an eight-inch kitchen knife, you get an all-inclusive trip to the wonderful and always sunny Sandals resort of mental illness. I approach his room and find him lying in bed, head turned to the right in a display of vivid hopelessness. Naturally, I walk to the right side of the bed to be in his line of sight. I introduce myself and begin to take stock of the situation. I plead with him to respond and to give me some semblance of regret for his suicide attempt. Instead, he turns his head to the left, never muttering a sound. I move to the foot of the bed and gently explain the process of an involuntary hold and the loss of freedom following inpatient admission.

"I can't determine that you're not a danger to yourself if you won't talk to me, Derek. I know you're suffering, but I am here to help. Can you tell me how you're feeling right now?" I receive no reciprocation of speech. He fails in an attempt to move his eyes from a fixed gaze.

He appears a beaten man, a case of human suffering from within. I make one final comment and let him know that I am going to send him to the mental health hospital for a few days to start some medications that may improve his symptoms. Again, he blankly stares at the tan curtain that divides this large room into separate and smaller areas of suffering. I can't imagine attempting to find health or sanity in a room shared with a stranger to whom you never speak and rarely see. Alone, you suffer in pain, and alone, a stranger suffers alongside you. No banter to each side and no speeches of motivation. You are singular, in a group of two, simply trying to remain positive regarding your outlook for recovery as you hear the moans of human agony only feet away. You are separated from the one you wish not to become only by a flimsy, tan-colored curtain. This curtain, however, represents the delineation of similarities between two souls in turmoil. Receiving no response from Derek, I proceed with the involuntary hold and have him admitted to the mental health hospital.

The next day, I find myself on call at the mental health hospital, and on my team is none other than the individual I committed the day before. I see Derek's name on my schedule and decide to see him first to verify the validity of my decision for admission, and of course check on his progress.

I hope I will find a young man seated at the edge of his bed reading quietly. I envision being greeted with pleasantries as he displays remorse for his actions of self-mutilation, followed by an in-depth talk about the brain and the mind as well as his mood and coping mechanisms. I hope we can even spend some time discussing medications or simply telling each other jokes, all as we laugh in dismantled pain now rebuilt with stability and progress. This, unfortunately, would not be the case today.

Making my way through the doors to the unit, I recognize many familiar faces, both of employees and patients. I tell the charge nurse that I am here to see Derek.

"He is in the day room," she responds.

I walk past the four windows looking into the day room and see Derek sitting at a table facing one of the windows to the courtyard on the farthest side of the room. He appears to have isolated himself to a position where he can be alone in his thoughts, stoic amongst the chaos around him.

As I approach, I witness him using the mental-health-hospital-issued crayons and fashioning the colors into something on a blank piece of paper. As I approach from behind, walking to the side of him, I glance down at his handiwork. He has created a rather grim display of shades of black with intermittent green scales. This hairless beast displays large canines with what appears to be red marks dripping from them, which I assume to be representative of blood.

"Hey, Derek. How are you doing?" In true fashion, he doesn't respond. In fact, he doesn't even appear to know I am present and seated across from him in our little art table. I immediately grab a piece of paper from my clipboard and, taking some of the remaining crayons in the box, begin to color my own portrait. This goes on for several minutes, just two people enjoying a weekend of coloring.

"Damn," I say, breaking the silence. "Mine sucks." I hold out the picture in front of me in an attempt to discern the landscape of interpretation. "Yours is pretty good. Who is that?"

With eyes remaining fixed on his paper, he finally makes contact with me. "It's Krell. He is a reptilian. He is always with me and we are ready to leave."

"Okay, very cool." Somewhat lost for words, I struggle to find the appropriate queries to assess his mental state yet not push him back into silence from outright interrogation. "How often do you see Krell?"

"Always," he replies, his hand busily creating a dark-brown background with large strokes of the crayon. The paper demands that one hand hold it in place as the violent blows of color meet the landscape behind this crudely drawn reptilian figure.

"Does he ever talk to you?" I continue to draw anything I can think of, simply to remain in his element. I look up briefly to notice the stark contrast of colors between the two canvases. I find the gray crayon and begin to add some darkness to my own photo, further cementing rapport and commonality of technique.

"No, he speaks through my mind."

"Does he ever tell you to do things?" I search for content of the hazardous symptom know as command auditory hallucinations.

"Sometimes I hear the devil."

"Does the devil ever tell you to do things?"

"Sometimes."

I realize I have to be more direct with my questions to find some pertinent information amongst his minimalist answers. "Does the devil ever tell you to hurt yourself?" His strokes of color quicken, beginning to clump from the coatings of multiple layers. He responds without words as I can see in the movements of his hand that I am reaching the level of questioning that instills stress. It could be that the voice inside his head is telling him not to respond, which happens quite often in patients suffering from similar symptoms.

I realize that he has shared all he is willing to and that best practice is to create no further stress this early in his treatment. I slowly get up, thank him for his time, and let him know I'm always here to talk to him should he have questions or concerns.

Patients such as Derek typically have perceptual disturbances in the form of auditory hallucinations. These hallucinations are often commanding or derogatory and sometimes can even be narrative. The fact that he is endorsing visual hallucinations is more on the rare side and not as common as those hallucinations of an auditory type.

If we truly could hear the voice of God and it sounded like an external bullhorn commanding us repeatedly to do things, how many of us could reject this persistent instruction day after day?

I often wonder why it is always God, Jesus, or even the devil. Why do delusions often include working for the FBI or CIA? Why do I never get the undercover operative from the local mall loss prevention team, or an undercover agent from the military's elite water purification corps? Why is there this typical affiliation with professions of such prestige? Why is it always a voice of such insurmountable importance? Why is it not the voice of that albino kid that sat next to me in third-grade math class?

There must be some inherent grandiosity associated with auditory hallucinations. It must be the mind's way of making sense of the bizarre by associating such symptoms to those of a higher power or purpose, all to satisfy the mind's search for meaning related to the voices that ought not be present. It's certainly more romantic to believe one is a direct vessel to God than to admit life has presented you with a brain bent on fraud, a brain inspiring whispers, mistaken identities, and a perception of reality built on lies. These lies are not those expressed by others, but are the deceptions conjured through interpretation by one's own mind. What a sense of deception one must experience when unable to trust what is seen, heard, and felt as obvious truths—when all these perceptions are possible gifts of a wooden horse by a Trojan army or a form of Judas trapped inside the mind shrouded in betrayal.

It takes nearly three months of severe medical intervention in the mental health hospital to get Derek to a level his family and I feel is safe for discharge. He is in no way healed, but he also isn't looking to empty his bowels onto the floor with a kitchen knife. His friend and confidant, Krell, has taken a well-deserved hiatus, and the devil and Derek are no longer on speaking terms. He simply is not improving any further, so we are forced to assume his current presentation is his new and unfortunate baseline.

Some patients, after a first break psychotic episode, find partial or total recovery. This sometimes lasts for years, and sometimes these vacations from insanity are greatly diminished in time, recurring persistently with each new stressor or each brief non-compliance with medications.

Derek's case is one I am able to follow. Four weeks after his discharge from the mental health hospital, he arrives in my county outpatient office. I have met his mother during a multitude of concerned talks, but this is the first time I meet his father. Derek's parents are divorced, and, in typical fashion, much effort, piss, and vinegar were dished out in order to win the primary custodial rights of the child. Derek's mother won that initial battle and reveled in the success for the first 18 years of his life. However, upon talking to his father, I learn that, once Derek fell ill with a mental disorder, he was quickly sent off to his father's house, never to hear from his mother again.

A woman who at first seemed so concerned with his welfare, now left her son in the hands of his father. Maybe she felt guilty of her inability to keep him safe. Maybe she felt ashamed, believing his disease to be something created by her, or maybe his mere presence was a constant reminder of the suffering she could not bear to face. One can only speculate on issues of neglect, and while Derek has never made mention of the abandonment, I can imagine it weighs heavily on his heart. This Derek is now an adult, but only by chronological age. He remains a child in measurements of abilities, insight, and capacity to care for himself.

By the time he is presented to my office, his previous stability, which more or less comprised of being mute while being in denial of plans to self-harm, has been preserved.

He arrives with his father, a man in his early fifties who is thin and small of stature but full of energy. Derek's father is attentive and seems to have stepped up in providing care. I now see who provided Derek with the jockey-like body type of a thin, short stature, weighing no more than eight stones. Derek's father, Tom, has a ranch at some distance outside of town, and this is where he and Derek reside. The ranch appears, by all description, to be a place where the solitude and limited external stimuli meld with the organic calm of nature providing freedom from the distractions of the city. The ranch is reported to be filled with lemon groves along with numerous avocado and pomegranate trees. Even the groves of fruit themselves add structure and balance to Derek's world as each is carefully placed in a row of consistency. Derek is lucky to have a father who provides a sanctuary of sorts, allowing the seeds of recovery and proliferation to flourish.

I meet Tom as he follows Derek into the room. Derek has little to say to me, but this is expected as he never was much for conversation. Derek finds the seat on the right and Tom takes up the only remaining seat directly across from me. I initiate conversation with Derek and little reciprocation is provided. I start in very easy with him, only asking the most generalized softball of questions. As the assessment progresses, Derek begins to become anxious with visible tapping of his hands and feet.

In a bid to remove the stimuli causing his anxiety, he becomes a human parrot. The moment his anxiety begins to cause his brain distress, he looks for a way out and finds it by repeating all my questions and mimicking my movements. This continues for a few rounds of questions, and I do my best to not start laughing, as his interpretation of me is rather spot on. Tom attempts to rationalize with Derek but receives the same treatment as I do.

The repetition of a person's words, phrases, and mannerisms, which is called echolalia, is certainly a feature of schizophrenia; however, in this case, I believe it to be more of a stress-reducing form of protection. I don't press or make much of his behavior as I want him to feel safe in his de-escalation technique. The rest of the interview is focused on gathering information through his father. His father details a rather uneventful month as well as the new addition to the family, a German Shepard mix that wandered onto their property. Without tags, this dog made a home of the ranch, and Derek has taken great interest in its well-being and has been rather instrumental in the dog's care. As the assessment closes, his father requests an explanation of an interesting new symptom. He states that

Derek has been endorsing the ability to hear colors and taste sounds. This description is that of a rare neurological condition called synesthesia. I am not overly concerned with this occurrence, and I try to also give Derek's father a decent explanation of such sensation overlap.

"The entire brain is a structured network of connections. Like synesthesia, many neurological disorders, including schizophrenia, have possible links to abnormal communication between brain regions. Therefore, it makes sense to me that some of his connections regarding senses may also be intertwined. We have recently done imaging of his brain, so I'm not concerned about anything more serious than the schizophrenia we are already treating. Just think of it as a manifestation of his schizophrenia."

I'm not sure if his father understood or simply just gave up asking questions so I'd shut up.

Tom responded, "Okay, I can see that. So . . . we shouldn't be worried."

"No, not at all," I say to reassure him.

I, unfortunately, am unable to assure myself; I simply wish for father and son to remain positive. You cannot reach improvement in life, nor health, without first envisioning it and believing in its possibility. Life has a way of conforming to your dreams, but only if approached with perpetual faith and a bit of healthy stubbornness.

Derek and Tom continue to visit me during my remaining six months of county clinic, and each meeting is filled with uneventful reports. The lack of occurrences is all I can hope for, as it is a great marker of stability. Derek continues to wander the fruit groves, tend to his furry companion, and spend a great deal of time playing video games. I am thankful that, in the time I spent with him, I never saw, or was told of, any exacerbations of psychosis. Derek's course of illness appears to be stable as of now, and sometimes just not getting worse is all we can ask for.

I never did discover if Derek began to engage in more social interactions or if he ever regained the presence of his former self. I do know that his progress and stability were made possible by the man he called his father—a father that dedicated all his time to providing his son with the tools and environment for success through stability. Even with all the previous incidents in Derek's course of illness, he was one patient that I never had to worry about. I knew his father would always be by his side, and because of this, Derek was one of the lucky ones.

I remember our last meeting before my planned exit from that particular county. Tom reached across the table and shook my hand, thanking me for all the help I provided his son. In response, I looked directly into his eyes, attempting to convey my sincerity, and simply thanked him for being such an amazing father. I told him I only wished more fathers had the love and dedication to their children that he had displayed for his son, a dedication bred not in a time of convenience but a time of desperation. Tom's eyes began to swell, as did mine, and we parted quickly so we could maintain our outward perception as strong, dry-eyed men.

CHAPTER 16

Mistaken Identity

"Some of the biggest cases of mistaken identity are among intellectuals who have trouble remembering that they are not God."
—Thomas Sowell

On day 4,007, I am at the gym, enveloped in my music of motivation as I find myself seated on the bicep curl machine. Unfortunately, this stimulus of inspiration is only serving the purpose of keeping my mind busy, as I'm not truly engaging any will to complete this workout, at least not with any sort of focused fury. Feeling drained by the day, I simply negotiate through the movement. I can't imagine any real growth is taking place. My only hope is that the small battle won of actually making it to the gym warrants the time away from other less painful tasks. I try to focus on the mantra that, "The only bad workout is the one that didn't happen."

When I was younger, hearing men complain of not wanting to go to the gym after a long day of work would result in an internal judgement of laziness. At that time in my life, I could find no good reason to miss the music of barbell plates rumbling or feeling the energy provided by being surrounded by people all with a similar purpose. Now hovering around 40 years of age, I understand this plight and often use this excuse for my own.

It is at this moment, as I am feeling sorry for myself, that my eyes begin to play a cruel joke. I see a patient from earlier in the day on the very treadmill in front of me. There she is, plain as day. She is wearing a blue top, similar to the blue hospital top I witnessed her wearing earlier in the day. The treadmill is facing me, and we lock eyes for just a moment until I look away, not wanting to make her feel uncomfortable. She looks happy. I take a few further, well-timed glances and see no underlying mental health issues bubbling up through the self. There is no apparent distress even to a well-trained eye. She is just a young woman enjoying an evening at the gym. As my brain begins to recognize the mind's misstep, I realize, sadly, it is not her.

The woman I treated earlier in the day was a 32-year-old schoolteacher struggling with the onset of schizophrenia over the previous three years. The culmination of the illness robbed this influencer of children from her beloved career. The draining of self-fulfillment and free will was replaced with command auditory hallucinations, which taunted her with thoughts of self-harm and were often laced with derogatory content. I feel sad knowing that the patient from earlier in the day will most likely never be the joyful and vibrant lady on the treadmill in front of me.

Unfortunately, this is not a rare occurrence, as it is something that happens more and more as I progress through the years of watching bright souls dim. I see my patients in crowds and in the faces of unsuspecting people that cross my path.

It's the humanity in the patients you learn to search for so you may see the wholeness they once possessed and appreciate the person trapped within the illness. With this urge for clarity, however, comes the stubborn habit of relating all people to your patients, seeing each person as having the opportunity for lunacy and normalcy. It's then the faces of others begin to meld, and with your supreme efforts at remission comes the opportunity for the mind to see your patients as you wish to see them: healed, happy, and walking amongst the backdrop of society, no different than any other individual.

I can only imagine that the mistaken identities of patients I have treated are the reflections of humanity witnessed in other persons. Maybe it is guilt for the ones that I cannot save that lingers and plagues my sense of reality. Faceless patients have become people to me. People with loved ones. People with vivid wants and dreams resonating within a light of hope, that for my patients has often altogether become absent. These people become a person who is a sister, mother, father, or brother. Some even become schoolteachers only recognizable in the face of a stranger.

CHAPTER 17

We All Scream for Oysters

WHITAKER

"A three-year-old was examining his testicles while taking a bath. 'Mom,' he asked, 'are these my brains?' 'Not yet,' she replied."
—Allan Pease

Today is day 4,045. I begin my fourth and final year of psychiatric residency. This moment, the last year of my role as indentured servant, is one I have been yearning for with the same angst of a 13-year-old boy reaching the front of the line of his favorite amusement ride. It is a ride he has spent weeks prepping for, a ride he stood in line for the better part of the day to experience, a ride that begins with tears, followed by screams, and ends in an exhaustive expression drawn out through every syllable creating a mix of pain and discomfort to the ear. It is the expression of success in accomplishment for something you enjoyed experiencing yet prayed for its quick end. I envisioned that fourth year would be that period in time when my intellectual competence would peak and solidify. This is the time for which the future seemed most bright and my once distant goal finally within reach. This moment, blissful in its recognition, would not be available for appreciation today, as for me, this day generates vastly different emotions.

I wake on this day to find it no different than any other. I am not congratulated with gifts during a champagne brunch, there are no balloons, and my morning is without even one splinter of spirited confetti floating down from the sky. Instead, I find myself walking alone in a barren, concrete fortress, laden with a plethora of poor life choices, unfulfilled opportunities, and histories of poor parental influence, all in a haze of substance abuse among its many hideaways. The breadth of psychosis in a facility such as this can be grand with vastly different variations between patients and their symptoms presented. On these days when we witness moments of psychotic, neural mishaps, we appreciate the complexity and delicate intricacies of the human brain. Those moments that allow us to peer into the end of the spectrum of mental illness are usually filled with views never imagined, and we are often wishful to never bear witness to such views again. This day would serve as a simple reminder every time I glance upon myself stepping out of the shower in full naked splendor. This day, although complicated by trauma, would provide an appreciation for all the parts I was born with that remain intact and whole. Even the mere thought of this day would make me shake my head in disgust, as if I had just sampled something foul, along with a faint yet distinct discomfort in my pelvic area.

I traverse through the maze of identical concrete hallways, each corridor just as boring and lifeless as the last. Only prisons, jails, zoos, and perhaps dungeons have indoor concrete walkways, void of any sense of luxury. Shit, even Walmart attempts some decency of comforts with flooring other than that of the dull, grey look of an unfinished surface. It is not until my morning voyage reaches the last web of walls that I hear the piercing screams of a man being tormented. I prep my tattooed, tattered, and overworked body for another day in the crisis stabilization unit, the happiest damn place in town—a place unique in the kingdom known as the county jail.

The shouts continue without interruption, so I attempt to mentally prepare for the shitstorm I'm about to endure. Unfortunately, I don't have my umbrella, and the weather this morning calls for grey skies, constant screams, and an unfortunately high likelihood of precipitation. When I say precipitation, I really mean bodily fluids, since urine, as well as feces, can be used as an offensive weapon in prisons and jails. As my steps slow, I see the cautionary yellow paint signifying the threshold of the simply incarcerated to the land of the misplaced mentally ill. After the historical closure of sanitariums, a large proportion of patients with mental illnesses are doomed to receive psychiatric care as criminals instead of as patients. No sooner does my size-12 boot cross this threshold do I hear Pepper, the head corrections officer.

"Just in time, Doc. We've got a fresh one for you." Pepper's tone has a hint of sarcasm, which I have grown accustomed to, paired appropriately with her "Good morning, it's Monday" smile.

"Good morning, Pepper, and how are you this fine morning?" I never did grasp the appropriate hierarchy of the corrections officers, but I assume it's similar to the police force or the military. I guess I should probably address them more formally, but they don't seem to mind first name identifiers. I continue, adding my own sense of sarcasm as it's a little early to kiss her salty ass just yet. "Yeah, I heard him calling for me. You got a name for the gentleman requiring services?"

"First name is Whitaker. Last name is . . ."

I tune this part out as his last name is not important to me in this setting of acute instability.

Pepper adds, "Can you see him and put him on medications . . . please?" She is clearly sending a request my way that implies the wish for me to simply "shut him up."

"Okay, let's go say hi. What's his location?"

John quickly yells out, "Safety cell A2." John is a new corrections graduate and still trying to impress his comrades. He's that pain-in-the-ass kid in the first row of math class, always blurting out the wrong answer, but doing so with such great confidence that I often wondered if he was correct.

We head into the bowels of the crisis stabilization unit and into the pod adorned with maximum security "safety cells." Here inmates are stripped of all items that they could use to harm themselves or others. With only paper scrubs, an easy-tear blanket, reading glasses, and maybe a book or magazine, the individuals are left in solitude to recover from any acute intoxication, recent suicidal ideation, or homicidal intent. I follow the officers as they guide me to his cell.

Each cell is fixed with a large, all-metal door. Each door has one window above a rather thin, horizontal slot. This slot is normally locked but can be opened to slide in a food tray or to cuff, and subsequently uncuff, prisoners during transfer. From a distance, I hear him screaming obscenities to any and all bystanders, as well as verbally confronting those manifestations derived in his bruised brain and misguided mind. His face is pressed up against the window as we approach. Once he notices the caravan, he promptly turns around and walks away from the window. The unit's background music, which had been his screaming, is abruptly and eerily silent.

I approach the cell and peer through the small window, slightly bending down to see appropriately. I find him, back turned, and his bare ass staring at me. His body is slightly hunched over and it's obvious he is working with both hands busily in the area of his crotch, which is something I have, unfortunately, grown accustomed to seeing.

Assuming he is busy in self-pleasure, I turn away to give him the privacy any person involved in self-stimulation would deserve, but I can't help but feel the oddity of timing for such an act. About thirty seconds into his frolicking, I listen to my intuition and decide to intervene. Ignoring the uncomforting view of a naked writhing body before me, I glance through the small window again.

"Whitaker. My name is Dr. McLaughlin. Can we chat for a minute?"

He continues with his business, occasionally moaning as he looks to the ceiling.

"Whitaker!" I again call out.

Busy into his work, he pays little attention to my silhouette, only momentarily peering just slightly over his shoulder, almost as to make sure the audience remains attentive. While awaiting his crescendo, I glance at the disposition of his cell. It's in obvious disarray, as expected, with food wrappers and book pages strewn throughout. As I study the state of clutter, I hear John.

"Damnit, Whitaker. Get dressed! The doctor is here to see you."

No sooner than John's commands cease do my eyes catch Whitaker's jail-issued glasses on the ground. All the thoughts in my mind go silent. Even as I document this event months later, I notice a new onset of discomfort from my wooden chair and witness goosebumps on my arms as I type. Through the distractions, I make out that his state-issued glasses appear to have been broken. One lens appears cracked and the other lens is missing entirely from my view. I start to think of what this other lens could be used for. I call out to him again, with a request to talk. Just then, I see small drops of substance dripping between his legs. I notice the dark red tinge of this abundantly available fluid, and I quickly step back. Just then it all hits me.

"Get this door open! He's cutting himself!"

As soon as I finish my sentence, he turns to face the door in all his naked splendor. Blood is pouring from his crotch and beginning to pool on the floor, with the only adornment of his grey concrete foundation being a central drain; a drain that will come in handy today.

He stands calmly at attention with his hands hidden behind his back. This stillness of form is finally broken when his left hand begins to make its way into view, blood visibly and profusely dripping from whatever is held within his closed fist.

As John's nervous hands fumble the keys, he orders, "Cell A2 open! Open cell A2! I need backup!"

Just then the switchboard operator overrides manual control and remotely opens the door. As the door swings towards me, I step back just enough to feel the wind of the metal entrance brush my nose. The first officer jumps into the door well, and as he begins to negotiate for Whitaker to drop whatever he has in his hands, it is then that Whitaker's eyes meet mine. Looking straight at me, he smiles, knowing he won, knowing I could not stop what was about to happen. He took all the power I have as a physician and poured it down that damn drain, along with all the blood from his mutilated crotch.

As my eyes widen, he raises his left hand closer to his face and, with a quick acceleration through the last third of the movement, empties the contents of his hand directly into his mouth. He then leaves his mouth open to display the pearl in the oyster he has found, allowing me just enough time to dedicate to memory the view of a man's testicle, cut fresh from his body, now resting on his tongue. Just then, he suddenly shuts his mouth and, to my dismay, swallows. Things then slow down, almost as if my brain forcibly slowed reality to allow my mind the time to process the trauma I have just witnessed. I see the blood-stained hand pattern painted over his mouth, similar to Native American war paint. It is then that reality abruptly hits me. He just swallowed his own testicle.

"Get the fuck in there!" I exclaim loudly in a commanding voice, not realizing the little weight I carry in this facility that likens my command to more of a suggestion.

As the posse of corrections officers rush into the cell, he again shocks me. He does not move, he does not step back, and he doesn't even try to guard himself from the blow about to come. He just stands upright and laughs. This guy just cut a testicle out of his own scrotum and ate it, and now he is laughing with an impending clubbing on the horizon. The laughing quickly ceases as the officers force him to the ground and shackle his arms behind him. The shackling is followed immediately by a persistent scream. I'm not sure if it was from the concrete takedown, the tautness of the handcuffs, or the anesthetic of psychosis wearing off and exposing the true pain of his amateur, surgical handiwork.

It takes the emergency physician some time to confirm what I already knew to be true. Status post some heavy sedatives and an examination at the local emergency department, we learn that his operation was definitively one of self-mutilation with ingestion. In other words, he successfully cut open his scrotum and continued to free his right testicle from its organic constraints, taking hold of it with his left hand and swallowing it, ingesting it willfully as one would swallow a raw oyster.

Later that morning, after the screams and wails subside, after the blood is washed away, Whitaker is nestled soundly in his hospital bed. I take a quick moment to find respite in a simple chair facing a wall. As I sit, I replay the morning occurrence in my mind, trying to make sense of such an act. I attempt to explore the event rationally and quickly determine that this episode of psychosis is simply that. This simple definition is all I truly have to offer at this time. He is a man tortured by mental illness and solitude; a man left alone with only the voice in his head to accompany him. With each moment, the voice is gaining strength and influence upon his will. Intellectualizing the situation will certainly end in the conclusion that the mind is powerful and fragile at the same time. Applying logic will most certainly not indemnify his scrotal sack of its physical loss.

Honestly, despite the horrific nature of what just happened, I can't help but be slightly impressed. I mean, I'm appalled overall, but at the same time, I am a little intrigued and impressed. I'm not entirely sure I could successfully duplicate this surgical procedure even with anesthesia, a scalpel, and appropriate gauze to keep the area properly visible, and I'm a physician.

It wasn't until the following week, day 4052, that I had the opportunity to speak to Whitaker. It is only then that I began to uncover the depth and historical timeline of his psychosis. Of course, he has been intermittently refusing the medications I have prescribed for him. Even with only sporadic adherence to medications, Whitaker is visibly calmer and, most importantly, not screaming. His thought process appears to be somewhat improved, yet he continues to respond outwardly to internal stimuli (chatting with entities only he can hear or see), but with that of lessened severity and frequency. His inability to converse coherently has amended somewhat but remains a barrier to full rational speech. Basically, he is still severely sick. Although improved in comparison to our previous encounter, I will require a creative approach with him to gather any viable data.

My mind begins to question the appropriate place to start our conversation. What do I say to a man that, only seven days ago, was screaming uncontrollably and eating his own testicle? Maybe if I don't bring it up, he won't, and we can just pretend it didn't happen. I'd certainly love to forget it ever happened. I'm sure he would as well. No! I can't just forget it happened; he swallowed his damn testicle, for God's sake. That's not something you just overlook.

What do I say? "Hi, Whitaker. Have you lost weight?" Maybe, "Hey, man, you know what they say, one less testicle, one less problem."

After a thorough introduction, I begin the conversation with the most obvious of questions: "Whitaker, last time we met, you did something very disturbing. I'm curious if you remember what I'm referring to?"

Gesturing to his crotch, he replies, "Yeah, I remember."

"Well, you were obviously suffering, and I can understand wanting to relieve some of the pain in any way necessary, but why did you mutilate your genitals?"

"Voices in my head. They don't stop. I ain't no fag! I showed them."

I evaluate his facial expressions and the painful memories bubbling up from his core. I hear his foot begin to tap the floor with ever-increasing speed, matched with an increase in rocking back and forth. I determine this may not be the best time to dig deep into a most recent traumatic event. Instead, I slow down the conversation and attempt to garner some historical insight by just letting the conversation progress naturally. I let his outward emotional expressions set the tone of the interview.

His psychosis remains present and florid, indicating a possible underlying primary psychiatric disorder with psychotic features. The seven-day washout period during his incarceration lessens the chance his current psychosis is merely secondary to substance intoxication. A negative urine drug screen in the emergency room last week confirms my suspicion. Here psychopharmacology trumps intensive psychotherapeutic techniques with the primary goal being medication-induced remittance of psychosis.

Blurring and entangling all that is perceived as reality, Whitaker's psychosis makes a meaningful conversation consisting of good-ol' fashioned logic very difficult. I need to gain his trust as we move forward in order to create a positive therapeutic relationship—a relationship wherein he sees me as someone he can confide in. Trust is difficult to gain in any person, especially after only one or two sessions; however, this case is further complicated by paranoia and insanity.

The assessment, while painfully long, eventually uncovers a five-year history of symptom manifestations. Struggling through the details of his past, we first must overcome great difficulty in finding a linear timeline of events. His memory, just as his reality, is fragmented, all merging into one wild ride. Finally, we both catch the same wind in our sails traveling in parallel down memory lane. Using key dates from his past, I am able to give his memory a springboard of reference. Through this direction, we explore initiation of symptoms, as well as the content of those symptoms, all of which surround significant reference markers throughout his life. This is a way to provoke his recall for a finite moment while calming his presently disrupted thought process. We all have difficulty remembering our state of emotional health for some random day in the past; however, most of us will be able to recall details and emotions on our first day of high school, our first kiss, our driver's license test, or our prom.

Whitaker describes voices—auditory hallucinations—starting at the age of 14, during his freshman year of high school. This is interesting as it is actually a bit earlier than most people with schizophrenia. These perceptual disturbances began as innocuously as hearing his name being called when no one was present. Being a freshman in high school, with much larger social issues to address, he simply wrote it off as of little importance, until it began to occur at home in the presence of solitude.

Over the years, this singular male voice would become multiple, and with the different voices would come different auditory experiences. The harmless voice calling his name eventually gave way to alternative voices, some of which were derogatory and persecutory in nature. His most distressing voice originated somewhere in his senior year of high school and involved the voice of a father figure emasculating him.

The voice would often utter, "You're nothing. No one likes you. You're not a real man."

This voice was persistently striking all of his actions and thoughts with dissatisfaction and perpetually questioning his role as a man. He describes living in a constant state of uneasiness. This relentless mistreatment, by what was perceived to be a father figure, may have very well been created or exacerbated by mistreatment from his own father. This is, however, not something we can explore at this time as he is already facing traumatic recollections from his past, and I have no wish to take him further down the rabbit hole.

Sometimes the mind will construct delusions atop hallucinations to make sense of such intrusions. Often the mind will look for the path of least resistance; therefore, it is possible that rather than facing the pain of constantly disappointing this father-like voice, he developed the delusion that the voice was that of an ever-present alien. Yes! I said aliens. As in, some other-worldly entity, misguided and bent on the destruction of everything Whitaker.

As ridiculous as this may sound, to Whitaker, this gave a path to understanding and a way to reason with the disappointment voiced. This belief provided him a sense of relief, since the voices were from aliens and were completely out of his control. He didn't have to contemplate if his brain was ill, nor did he have to give credence to the derogatory voice of an alien. Whitaker's mind was right, as these voices were far from the reach of his influence, and they were certainly alien to his mind. Unfortunately, these aliens were not from a distant galaxy, nor had they traveled through a wormhole; they simply occurred as a product of a biological illness inside his brain. This predisposition to such illness was most likely genetically passed along to him, possibly activated through some environmental stressor, be it drugs or trauma or even due to a hereditary inclination of synapses to "over-pruning" in the developing adolescent brain.

Whitaker's accounts continue, and from what little he provides, I can make generalized assumptions. From what I gather, depression began to set in throughout his high-school years, and with it, isolation and an increased conglomeration of what are considered negative symptoms. These "negative" symptoms are so called because of the visible loss of normal social responses and cues to human interactions they create. With their representative loss of humanistic behaviors, a person begins to form behaviors and interactions likened more to a featureless robot than that of a person. People with schizophrenia may present with limited emotional affect, blank looks, monotone speech, a lack of interest in the world, and an organic inability to feel pleasure. These negative symptoms are often the most difficult to treat and are often reported by patients to be the most debilitating. Patients with schizophrenia are often forced to suffer locked inside a mind that feels no pleasure, has no motivation to speak or interact. They often remain imprisoned in an existence free of all the emotional qualities that define our humanity.

Aside from these negative symptoms, a person with schizophrenia can also experience depression. Depression most often occurs in people with higher cognitive functioning prior to illness. It's as if just enough of the self remains to realize what has been lost and what goals and aspirations will never be realized. Positive symptoms, such as hallucinations and delusions, are, for the most part, easier to treat. Due to the often concerning and frightening disposition of positive-type symptoms, they have become the most frequent reason patients with schizophrenia seek, or are provided, treatment. These positive symptoms are the ones that lead family members to seek urgent assistance.

Whitaker endorsed a lack of friends or participation in extra scholarly activities throughout high school, and with such lack of social supports he most likely fell into a state of self-excommunication. As high school progressed, so did his illness and his quarantine from society. The alien in his head became the only being he had to converse with or confide in. The alien knew all his secrets and his weaknesses. It presented as taking great pleasure in exposing his frailties. This anxious boy became a defenseless and disheveled man of 19 years of age.

Per his accounts, there was a time when his parents sought out help and were able to secure psychiatric care from a county clinic for adults. At this time, Whitaker was prescribed an extensive cocktail of medications that soon began to display effectiveness in his mood and thought, leading to decreased isolation. The medications continued to prove efficacious, creating a generalized remittance of nearly all his symptoms.

According to Whitaker, "It was like someone turned down the T.V. in my head."

Over the next six months, his symptoms continued to diminish. With this temporary remission of symptoms came the idea that the necessity for psychiatric medications was unfounded. Along with the coercion of his family, he decided to abruptly discontinue his regimen, believing his previous incident to be nothing more than outliers from his baseline level of function. This was most likely a moment of great relief for his parents, as they could convince themselves that their son's psychosis was just a "phase." It was the conclusion that they wanted to believe.

Unfortunately, when his illness boiled over again, it came back with a vengeance. Although his parents swiftly recanted their previous position and urged for medication adherence, the voices inside his head were too ingrained and would relentlessly counter all attempts at compliance.

"You don't need medications! They are trying to change you. They are trying to poison you. Just say you took them, no one will know."

This is a common theme for many patients with schizophrenia, and this is exactly what Whitaker describes. This time, the voices were no longer sitting idly by. They were bent on destruction with self-preservation near the end of their list of goals and objectives. The voices were the puppeteer and Whitaker was a wooden boy, attached to strings. Being pulled in every which way, he was led out of the protection and comfort of his parent's home. He found sanctuary on the streets, where he could roam and converse with himself without the watchful eyes of discerning people. Months passed, and with each new moon, the persistence of his illness engulfed, bit by bit, everything he once was.

He would catch the attention of a store owner one day, which prompted a call to the police. Disorderly conduct was the charge. Apparently, being naked while yelling at customers as they walk into a restaurant is frowned upon.

Once in custody, screaming and yelling persisted, guiding his way into the psychiatric unit. I'm unable to determine if his constant yelling was a product of response to the voices or simply a device to drown them out.

The derogatory nature of Whitaker's auditory hallucinations did not relinquish or relent during incarceration. They continued to emasculate and humiliate him. Over time the voices took the more ominous form of commands suggesting self-harm. These perceptual disturbances would encourage him to kill himself to ease the burden on his family; often expressing the idea that he should just cut his dick off if he wasn't going to use it. "No woman would ever want you. You're a pussy! You're a ball-less pussy!" Eventually, his only escape from his own mind was to follow the commands, hoping that once the voices were satisfied, they would return to the dark hole or planet they came from. This is where his motivation for self-injury arose, and part of me can almost understand why he did what he did. His act of cutting out a testicle was his way of saying, "Here! Is this what you really want?" It was almost like it was evidence of strength, a slap in the face to those voices that doubted his resolve.

At our next meeting, I decide to try my hand, one more time, at determining the source of this derogatory male voice. Its predominance makes me wonder if this had been an inner dialogue derived from some previous trauma. I sit with him during our typical Wednesday meeting. It is like most of our other meetings, except that this time I have an intern shadowing me. I ask Whitaker about his father and provide him with my reasoning for such questioning. He responds in denial but gives reasons contradicting such denial.

"No, my dad never really said mean things to me. He probably thinks I'm a loser, and I could just tell he was always disappointed in me." In a brief moment of clarity, the words come out of his mouth effortlessly, as if to repeat a consistent thought. Then, just as quickly, his defenses are hoisted back up. Again, the mind is filling in gaps for things that have no validity of concept, ideas too scary to embrace as truth. His mind returns to delusional rationalizations. "I know it's aliens. It's always those fuckin' aliens!" He begins to pace back and forth in his cell, whispering to himself.

"Whitaker, I want to prescribe you some new medications." Trying to refocus his attention, I present this to him with a soothing tone, offering some relief from his suffering through psychopharmacology.

"Meds don't work, Doc. I ain't taking meds!"

"No problem, man, I get it." I offer thanks for his time as I pretend to leave the area, stepping out of his view, if only for a second, to garner some dramatic essence.

"Whitaker. Hey, Whitaker, come to the window. I want to tell you a secret." He stops dead in his tracks and walks over to the window. As he approaches, I look over my left shoulder and quickly follow it with a glance over my right shoulder, acting with a sense of nervousness about what I'm about to tell him. I lower my voice to continue this perception and lean in close to the window. "I have a medication that helps with aliens."

"What? Really?"

Further thickening the plot, I add, "Yeah, man, but you can't tell anyone. It's on the down-low. I'll start it today just for you. Okay?"

"Hell yeah, man! Thanks, Doc." He confirms his willingness to try this untested, off-label use of antipsychotics.

For now, I'll let the anti-alien medication work its magic, decreasing the overabundance of dopamine in Whitaker's fragile brain. I hope next week we can have a much more natural conversation, and I look forward to meeting the man beyond the mental illness.

As we walk to the dictation room, the intern shadowing me that day reluctantly asks me a question. He had been out of Whitaker's visual field yet within range to hear the entire conversation.

The intern cautiously inquires, "Doctor, can I ask a question?"

"That depends. If you are going to ask me about a personal issue like a rash or burning on urination, then no. Anything else is fair game."

"It's about when you told him you had a medicine for aliens. Are we supposed to play into or engage them in their delusions?"

"Nope!" I quickly answer. "But sometimes, I do. It's all about your intentions. If your intentions are pure, then your only goal should be to help the patient in any way you possibly can. If I can help him by telling him this medication may be effective against aliens, and if I can get him to buy into the necessity of treatment, then maybe, just maybe, we can find a window of clarity and a way to reach him in a more lucid state."

I continue on. "I do things a tad different than most psychiatrists. We are not supposed to improvise. We are not supposed to share things about ourselves or our personal lives with our patients, but I do. You have to know when it's appropriate. I sometimes will provide small details of my own history to add relatability, but only when I believe it's going to positively affect treatment, help establish trust, and secure the therapeutic relationship. If a situation meets all such criteria, then I feel the benefits are worth the risks. I think it's absurd that we feel we have the right to ask our patients about sexual orientation, history of abuse, suicide attempts, etcetera, yet when they ask something about us, most psychiatrists hide behind their perceived cloak of superiority, getting their panties all bunched up at the thought of answering a simple question. Just decide who you want to be. You can be the psychiatrist that does exactly what he was told to do by a bunch of old outdated dusty opinions, or you can just be yourself and allow your personality and your experiences encourage the relationship you build with your patients. Don't be afraid to push against the system a bit. Nothing changes without a little force. Remember, there are two types of medicine. One is the practice of 'classroom medicine' in its sterile confines of a textbook or in a simulation room, complete with predetermined scenarios. The other world of medicine is found in the actions of 'clinical medicine,' which takes place in the real world, a world with patients that scream, bleed, swallow testicles, and sometimes try to kill you!"

CHAPTER 18

Light My Fire

BRANDY

"It's funny how everyone hates witch hunts . . .
until they see a witch."
—Jon Stewart

Sometimes there is simply a need to light people on fire! That is the concept Brandy struggles to convince me of on day 4,082. Her conviction is certain and her belief solid. It's possible that under different circumstances, and through a more reliable vessel, I may be persuaded to partially agree to such a misguided notion. However, in this reality, which she and I do not completely share, I reserve my right to judgment.

Today I find myself in the county jail, but not as an inmate, so that's an encouraging start for the day. Before meeting Brandy, I find myself in recovery trying to calm the beast inside, yet still writhing from the surge of adrenaline brought on by the patient preceding her. I prefer to have my morning spike of catecholamines be due to elevated quantities of ingested caffeine. Unfortunately, I have had little time to bring the liquid, filtered through roasted seeds—yes, they are seeds, not beans—to my lips.

Nothing says "good morning" like a conversation with a 55-year-old male awaiting sentencing for rape and imprisonment of a child. This predator squandered what little time I granted him, not requesting help for his inner demons but trying to win my sympathy for his incarceration. Often inmates have this idea that somehow the prison doctor can sway decisions of the gaffe. This is simply not true. We are two separate entities of the system, with two unique duties. Our authorities, however, are also unique. As a psychiatrist, my power is limited to those troubles of medications and inmate safety. I may also be afforded the ability to make recommendations regarding other matters, but the judge has the true power in this kingdom. Regardless of how many times I explain this to the patients before me, they persist in their stories of innocence, holding onto hope that if they act appropriately with me, convincing me of their virtue, I will somehow whisper into the judge's ear, coercing his decision.

His story—and I rightly label this as a story, or better yet, a fable—was that the sex he had with a 13-year-old girl was not the fault of his but laid solely on the shoulders of the underage girl. This did well to spark the repugnance inside me. I felt as though an ammonia inhalant had just been cracked under the nose of my repressed anger. An incident attempting to evoke a response from the conventional reaction I have hidden well behind the wall of professionalism. My pulse quickened, and I can only guess the Irish side of my descent was a fiery glow, represented by the addition of a bright-red hue to my face. All courtesy of his statements detailing the entire episode in question as the product of her initiation. Forged fabrications continued, asserting the child as the perpetrator of dirty deeds and labeling himself as the victim of rape, all while he was helplessly passed out after a night of binge drinking.

As our time, and my fuse, came to an end, I looked at him and leaned my torso into his space. This was not just any lean but a lean that was over-exaggerated, intentional, and that to provide a most uncomfortable distance for him. In a quiet voice, I uttered to him, "Is this really the story you're going to give in court? Good luck with that!" Shaking my head, I led him out the door and back into the hands of deserved custody.

I close the door and sit motionless in my chair, simply staring at the wall ahead of me. Proud of myself for remaining relatively calm, I try to decompress and quiet the disgust bubbling up inside. This type of repulse can only be caused by being in the presence of evil—the pungent flavor of evil that can attempt justification, or even an excuse, for the rape of a child. It's sickening to think how he extinguished the purity and joy that should accompany youth, all for a moment of projected power and orgasmic pleasure. Forever gone is her innocence, and no sentence, nor amount of incarceration, will ever grant restoration to the victim.

I remain disposed within the office chair, contorted in complacency, for whatever position my body chooses. My face embraces respite within my hands as I begin to feel ill in the discouragement of defeat due to the frequent witness of my species' primitive acts and entitlement to urges.

I'm slightly startled when the door swings open. A voice shouts, "We got another one for you! This is Brandy. Brandy, say hi to the doctor." I lift my head out of my hands, stand from my chair, and turn to the door. I'm about to forcibly tell them to give me five more minutes until I see a young woman in four-point restraints. My curiosity overcomes the now simmering fury.

The restraints attach each of her limbs to its own metal bracket. Each bracket is welded to the wheelchair she is being transported on. She is adorned with a bright orange jumpsuit, chains around both legs and wrists, all attached to a singular long chain that is further affixed to her waist. This metal jail-house bling forces a mild hunched-over posture as the chain from her hands to her feet is slightly shorter than would allow full upright posture. To further complicate this metal sudoku, she has a second pair of handcuffs attached to her wrist to further restrict her ability to break loose. All she is missing is the classic Hannibal Lecter mask. For some strange reason, I think to myself, *How great would it be if she is a forensic psychiatrist with a European accent and a sophisticated palate for fine chianti?*

The guards help her out of the chair by releasing all four restraint points, and with one guard on each side basically lifting her out of the chair, they escort her to the corner of my office. Here there is a plastic chair just free-floating and next to it a wooden bench affixed to the wall and floor with two separate points of adhesion. They sit her on the wooden bench and cuff her leg chain to the large metal bracket sunk into the concrete flooring.

"That's not necessary, guys."

"Sorry, Doc, with this one we have to. Order from above, ya know?"

I understand the illusion of hierarchy, so I don't push the issue. I realize there is probably a big stack of paperwork they would have to fill out if this lady successfully chewed off my face and wore it as a mask.

As the guards find their way out of the room, one turns to me. "We will be right outside if you need anything."

Trying not to laugh, I respond, "I think we will be okay." I note the small frame of the woman shackled and chained to the floor like a wild animal. "Hello, Brandy. It's nice to meet you. My name is Doctor Mclaughlin and I'm a resident psychiatrist."

She just laughs, looking at me while giggling and trying to squirm in her chair as if to use the metal clanking as some sort of mating signal. "Ah, they knew what I like; they are setting me up. I love me white boys with blue eyes."

"Okay, so how are you feeling today?"

"Oh, I'm good now," she says while smiling, giggling, and continuing to squirm in her chair like a nervous high-school girl.

"Brandy, can you tell me why you're here?" As I slightly turn my body towards the computer, I quickly scan her initial admission note from the therapist tasked with documenting the overnight admissions. I read the sentence, "Two counts attempted murder. Blunt force trauma. Lit both biological parents on fire as they sat on the couch watching television. Extinguished by adult brother and brother-in-law, both in the house at the time of the incident."

"I have no idea why I'm here."

"Did something happen at home with your parents?" I ask.

"My family are witches!" she screams. "They practice witchcraft. I can see that now."

"Oh, okay." That is the only response I can come up with as I attempt to maintain composure. "When did you start having these thoughts? What I mean is, the thoughts that your family members may be witches." I am trying to clarify the onset of symptoms, or at the very least, this particular symptom.

"I have always felt different from my family, and then I realized why. They are damn witches! Witches! Witches! Witches!"

"Tell me how you know."

"Well, one time my uncle was at the front door and then the cops drove up and he disappeared. Next time I saw him he was at the back of the house. It was so quick that the only way he could have got back there is if he flew over the house. Sometimes I'll be talking to my mom and it's not her; I can tell it's my aunt. Sometimes when I'm talking to my dad, I can tell it's not him, it's my mom. They think I don't know but I figured it out. I figured all their shit out."

Brandy continues to explain that her family members have the ability to trade bodies and "shape-shift." Subsequently, on one occasion, she became frustrated with the shifting of consciousness and decided to force her mother and father to return to their original bodies by pouring gasoline on them and lighting them on fire.

"I wasn't trying to hurt them; I was just trying to make them switch back. Fire is the only way to do that. You can't kill them that way. I don't know why everyone is making such a big deal of it. They use witchcraft, so they can't be killed that way." She speaks in a matter-of-fact approach, with an attitude as if to infer this is common knowledge.

At that point, she looks away and begins a conversation with someone only she can see.

"Shut up! I'm trying to talk to him. It's not the same guy. Oh, what do you know? You don't even know him!"

"Do you want to introduce me to who you're talking to?" I ask.

"I'm not talking to anyone," she declares in a paranoid state as she lowers her shackled arms close to the floor and places her head against one leg. With her mouth facing away from me, she continues to converse with this most intrusive of confidants. She whispers, hoping I won't hear the secretive conversation taking place before me. The gossips become louder as the conversation continues, leading to a crescendo outburst. She quickly stands up; the multiple thick chains connecting all her limbs indirectly to a wooden chair loudly clank together.

"Shut the fuck up or I'll kill you!" she voices loudly, still talking to the air.

The guards outside the door quickly open the only exit. I put up my hand, gesturing to hold their entrance. At this point, she grabs hold of this invisible entity and brings it to the floor as if she is in a real-world confrontation. Flailing her fists at what undoubtedly is the entity's head, she screams out, "I'll kill you! I'll fucking kill you!"

No strikes are actually hitting the ground, and aside from the scene, nothing is disturbed or physically damaged, so I allow this barroom brawl to play its course. I softly, but sternly, call out her name as to distract her from the beat-down she is currently involved in, and dishing it out quite well, I must add. Hearing me call her name, she quickly becomes uninterested in her foe, abruptly stopping the engagement as she sits back down slowly on the wooden throne. She adjusts her nonexistent hair with a few quick shakes of her head. Her lack of hair, most likely the result of a fresh homemade hack job, doesn't seem to trouble her. She brushes her imaginary hair to the side with her hands, still shackled for what I'm now assuming is her own protection. She looks up at me and we meet in a smile.

"Sorry about that," she said.

"What just happened?" I ask.

She gives no response other than falling into a child-like giggle, covering her mouth with what her hands could reach.

"I don't know," she says in a high-pitch and long, drawn-out course, accentuating each syllable as would a shy child when asked what his or her favorite toy is.

Who was this unseen figure and what did it represent? Often those perceptual disturbances involving people are symbolic, the figure encompassing a period of stress, trauma, or suffering. Yet, with her current level of disorganization, I realize there is little to be learned with a lengthy assessment. No curtains of clarity will be opened today. I know not if her psychosis is due to that of a brief psychotic episode induced by substance use or a form of something much more ominous, such as schizophrenia. I move towards antipsychotic treatment options and devise a plan to address her psychosis. In configuring a plan for Brandy, her current state complicates an accurate verdict. Therefore, I move to the only tool in the toolbox that I can currently identify a need for. I choose a hammer of psychopharmacology. While I cannot confirm her diagnosis, nor the reason for her symptoms, I do what I can. From this acceptance, I find comfort in the dark and simply treat the symptoms.

As a psychiatrist, I am often nothing more than a spectator watching illness unfold. The witnessed responses in settings of visual hallucinations allow me to gain an impression regarding the world of psychosis. Yet, with the very little historical data I have on Brandy's past, it's difficult to gain a solid perspective on what that current entity encompasses or represents. New-onset visual hallucinations may also be due to deviations in intracranial processes, meaning they may be produced by seizures, brain lesions, or tumors. With this knowledge, if such manifestations continue to occur, one may be inclined to order neuroimaging to rule out acute or chronic intracranial processes, followed by an EEG to rule out a seizure disorder.

As I formulate a differential diagnosis, I have to think broadly for possible causes. I need to rule out substance-induced psychosis, brain tumor if new onset is a concern, blood levels, electrolytes, and even ergot poisoning. Yes, ergot poisoning is a real thing! I remember reading about the Salem Witch trials where some individuals credit the fungus Claviceps purpurea. This fungus, which affects rye, wheat, and other cereal grasses, has been pointed out as a potential instigator of madness. When first infected, the grains begin to sprout a flower, which releases a sweet nectar containing fungal spores. Eventually, the fungus invades the grain, turning the kernels of grain a purplish-black color. Often simply mistaken for discolored kernels of grain, these innocuous seeds contain potent chemicals. These powerful components, such as ergot alkaloids, including lysergic acid from which LSD is made, affect the central nervous system. This can lead to violent muscle spasms, delusions, hallucinations, and a mass of other symptoms, all of which are present in the records of the Salem witchcraft trials. It is a fitting cause to rule out, I figure, as this case also comprises of accused witchcraft. I guess it's a good thing we aren't in 1692 where such symptoms may have historically led to death by hanging or burning at the stake.

I give the dopamine suppression effects of risperidone time to calm her hallucinations and hopefully bring her mind back to a state of clarity, knowing well that its properties of sedation will acutely provide relief yet knowing the true downstream effects of such medications take time to reach maximum efficacy. Maybe complete clarity is a bit much to hope for. Let's try for improvement, with the initial goal of fragmented lucidity. The overall goal is to develop a situation in which Brandy and I can talk on concepts of reality rather than those of the paranormal.

Although I cannot pin down an exact diagnosis at this time, my treatment will most likely not change regardless; unless, of course, I believe her condition to be that solely of substance intoxication. I bid adieu to my new friend, or friends, and send her and her entity back to the cozy confines of her chamber. I hope to see her again in the very near future, with the expectation of improved circumstances.

This is one of the issues regarding psychiatry in the inpatient emergency department, as well as in correctional settings. Often, we see these patients and develop a sense of compassion and concern for their well-being, only to have follow-up care diverted to an outpatient provider or to that of the on-call psychiatrist via telemedicine. Additionally, as a resident physician, you never stay in one place for long, and therefore continuity of care is predictably absent. As a resident, you are forced to care for the individuals and then quickly move forward to the next patient, relinquishing all concern for your patient's future well-being. This is easy for some, while others find this unknown to be somewhat tortuous.

It is from the experience of meeting Brandy, amongst a multitude of unfortunate incarcerated souls, that I begin to question the usefulness, or better yet the proficiency, of the judicial system. Its purpose is obvious, but is it possible we could find a way to more rapidly differentiate those in need of psychiatric care, as to whether a symptom or reason for their legal discordance, from those with clear-minded discontent for the legal and moral statutes of society?

Since the deinstitutionalization of "insane asylums" in the 1950s, individuals with psychiatric disorders have been left to largely suffer on their own. Attempting to gain assistance in a system set with few inpatient beds, fewer mental health hospitals, and very little funding to build more infrastructure, individuals often are forced to forgo treatment. Many of those without treatment never regain the establishment of employment or housing, and if without family members, most will find their path leads to homelessness. If not homeless, they find involuntary refuge in crowded city and county jails. The jail is a violent place of incarceration and ultimately a much worse existence than that found in a prison. I always found this perplexing as jails often provide a place for individuals awaiting trial and prior to any conviction, yet the more humane treatment found in prisons is after the individual has been ruled guilty in conviction for his or her crimes. Jailing people with mental illness creates huge burdens on law enforcement, corrections, and state and local budgets. It does not protect public safety for the long term and only further excludes those individuals from an already thin bridge to help.

Initially, I assumed prison would present with the most complicated and trying cases for the psychiatrist; that was until I experienced both prison and jail. It was then that I determined that jails were the worse of the two. The overall instability of patients in their acute state along with the shock of recent incarceration without time to mentally adjust leads to the muddiest of mental states—states of the mind ruminating from its uproot of familiar settings, along with the stress of possible lengthy prison times. To add insult to injury, the high prevalence of drug intoxication or withdrawal is the perfect cocktail for the mentally ill to jump further into the pool of madness. Swimming in their psychiatric disorders, diagnoses are obscured by acute stress and substance use.

Although a psychiatrist would likely prefer a more stable setting, the jails and emergency rooms are the front lines of mental illness. The city and county jails may be the most challenging environments to work for the psychiatric resident physician. Still in training, the psychiatric resident is accustomed to the environment of the mental health hospital, the emergency department, and the outpatient settings, yet little can prepare him or her for the emotional torment commonly apparent in the jail. In a mental health crisis, however, people are more likely to encounter the police than a medical professional. Therefore, to truly study and prepare for all environments, the psychiatrist-in-training should at the very least have some exposure to the mentally ill hidden behind those walls.

CHAPTER 19

Polarity Unrestrained

ANNA

"The statistics on sanity are that one out of every four Americans is suffering from some sort of mental illness. Think of your three best friends. If they are okay, then it's you."
—Rita Mae Brown

I find myself at my desk and looking up at my alarm clock. It taunts me as it reads 11:45 pm, and it does so with cheap, red neon numbers, which I'm sure were all the rage in the 1980s but have now been deemed as a useless trinket by today's standards. Although it's late, I have just finally caught up with work-related documentation and other duties surrounding persistent residency requirements. I feel the exhaustion as I find myself in a struggle of determination and stubbornness with my own eyelids. My poor attempts to squint and maintain focus have led to severe discomfort in my vision, all secondary to an internal struggle to function without glasses, for which I'm nearly certain I require. I struggle to find the energy during this process of medical residency.

Through these late hours, I reflect on the patients I have treated. I pour through the ever-growing stacks of notes detailing patient encounters, typically word for word as they occurred. It is then I notice that the only notes considered to be incomplete are those related to patients suffering from acute episodes of mania. It's not for a lack of potential patient stories but a simple deficiency of recorded dialogue.

The patients in manic states have elevated moods and speech that is rapid and pressured. Often patients in an acute manic phase will talk with such feverish frequency that attempting to scribe their words becomes close to an impossibility. Aside from the aforementioned complexities, the subject of this rapid speech is oftentimes tangential in thought process, never returning to the original topic, and seeming to jump from ideas related to only the voice in which they are expressed. It is already difficult to properly dictate what was said during any patient encounter. Yet, with the manic patient, due to the sheer gravity of subject matters and elevated levels of vitality and drive, trying to put ideas verbatim on paper is nearly impossible.

I'm not certain if it's the lack of sleep or the complexity of bipolar disorder that creates tension in my fingers as I struggle to communicate an experience that can somehow shed light on the illness and its grand spectrum of diversity. One would be hard-pressed to find another psychiatric disorder with the ability to cause such discomfort and pure exhaustion in the provider.

We live in a misinformed culture in which people loosely use the word "bipolar" without any true sense of its framework. We hear, "I think she is bipolar because sometimes she is super nice and then suddenly, she can be a bitch!" This type of description is more in line with a person suffering from issues of mood lability, impulse control, or emotional dysregulation, all birthed by a multitude of factors, most of which are based in personality. It is also altogether possible that this person may simply be, in the derogatory sense of classification, someone possessing a disposition considered as "bitchy." Mood swings, impulsivity, and tumultuous relationships, while fitting of a designation of polarity, does not always equate to medically defined bipolar disorder. The literal definition of polarity does not truly encompass the distinct characteristics of bipolar disorder, nor does it come close to its presentment of severity and distinction.

I like to think of bipolar mania as an elevated cocktail of primary emotions, all created by an amateur bartender with no perception or appreciation for balance. It's like a concoction of elevated mood and subjective magnificence being wound up in an ill patient energized beyond all what is human. The manic patient has the unique ability to manipulate situations and outmaneuver those around them, often by utilizing verbal slander and personal attacks. All these assaults lead to a sense of uneasiness and self-doubt in the unprepared mental health provider.

The manic patient needs no sleep, food, or drink. These individuals are not bound by human, heterotrophic properties. Instead, they appear to obtain their endless energy via photosynthesis. They have a knack for survival, seemingly using only the most basic of properties such as oxygen and sunlight for fuel. They are high on life with chemicals flowing through their brain giving them the green light 24/7, consistently pacing and devising new plans of world domination. No need to stutter, yield, or even check the crossing lanes. Just barrel through the intersection because you are the smartest, best-looking person on the planet. You are a god, so what could go wrong?

Bipolar disorder is a disease that may be a curse for some and a blessing for others. In some patients, it may encompass both. Many great minds of the past suffered from such a disease in various forms of spectrum severity. If blessed with bipolar disorder type 2, you may suffer from episodes of depression, but at times, you may also experience hypomania. This is a form of mania which differs from the more severe type 1 designation. Along the spectrum of bipolarity, those suffering from hypomania, indicated as type 2, experience a condition of less intensity and shorter duration, and although these periods are easy to notice from peers and loved ones, they do not typically cause significant impairment in functioning that would necessitate mental health hospitalization. These hypomanic periods can lead to elevated energy, motivation, and frequent bursts of creativity. For many, the blessing of inspiration, euphoria, and elevated confidence can still be seen as a curse, as baseline levels of normalcy begin to feel like depression. These episodes of depression feel tragically bleak, often accompanied by hopelessness and suicidality.

The depression of bipolar disorder, regardless of the type, is one of the most difficult mood disorders to treat. Bipolar depression does not respond the same to antidepressant medications as unipolar depression, which most people would simply call depression. Having experiences of manic episodes only further cement the depressive phases as being insurmountable.

It's day 4,120, and my next patient is Anna. Anna is a thin, unassuming, yet quick-witted Hispanic woman in her early thirties. Anna often prefers playful banter to conversations having depth. She has difficulty stepping aside from her defenses of humor. She rarely feels comfortable facing the risk of judgement or the impending display of painful emotions should she continue along a path requiring recall and assessment of historical trauma. Anna is never one to embellish on her sexual conquests nor one to even allude to discussions regarding those of sexual nature.

Throughout our time together, I maintain an informal and nontraditional stance, which allows me to build a pleasurable, doctor-patient relationship with her. It is a relationship free of judgement, coupled with a heavy dose of calling her out on her inconsistencies. This allows her to feel comfortable with me, ever willing to keep the truth at the forefront of our conversations as a measure of mutual respect. This also serves as an indication of a connection with a parallel goal. Our goal is simple: we search for stability and an understanding of her illness, all as we concurrently attempt to break down her boundaries to vulnerability.

On this day, Anna presents oddly, carrying a much more elevated mood as she struts into the office. Her state, bordering on elation. Even her dress is altered, as her reserved clothing is replaced by an outfit leaving little to the imagination. As we converse, I quickly become aware that Anna is caught amongst a contest of wills between her manic and non-manic self. Never has she presented this way before. I know of her bipolar disorder and its representative mania via historical criteria, but I have never seen her in such a state. Her speech is rapid and pressured. Her thoughts race from one topic to another, with no yielding for normal breath counts and providing little relevance to the original topic posed. This is worrisome as she appears to be nothing but a passenger of her own frenzied drive. Having had her as a stable patient for months prior to her current presentation, I am unprepared for this state of rapid decompensation.

All topics guided by her are those of sexual innuendos or reports of recent sexual conquests. As much as I try to steer this love bus of sorts, I am simply spoken over. It is as if my words warrant an objection from an opposing attorney, retained to allow only topics that are erotic in nature. The unassuming woman I have become accustomed to is on hiatus, and filling in for her is a shell guided by lower brain functions and primitive desires.

As I reflect on this experience, I clearly remember how the conversation began. "Nineteen," she states as she walked into my office, head held high as if she just won some sort of lifetime achievement award.

"Please tell me that's how many miles you walked or how many hours you spent gardening."

"Nineteen different partners this month."

"Nineteen different men?" I ask in complete shock.

"Well, they weren't all men," she says with a laugh.

"Okay." I pause to calm my disbelief and to hide any facial expression that could be construed as disgust. "Please tell me what is going on."

"I'm just bored and having fun," she adds, as calm as if I had asked her what she had eaten for breakfast.

"Okay . . . how is your sleep?"

"About two or three hours a night, sometimes zero. I don't really need sleep. I feel great. Shit! I drove to Texas last week on no sleep. I just drove straight there."

"That's over a thousand miles. What happened that made you want to drive to Texas?"

"Nothing, I just wanted to visit an old friend. I got the idea at night, and I couldn't get it out of my head, so I just left to visit him."

This back-and-forth charade continues without interruption for the better part of an hour. With every moment of conversation and detailed excursions, I become further shocked by the contrast of her current presentation with that of prior meetings. It leaves me feeling more like her father than her psychiatrist. I can't tell if she is being taken advantage of or if she is the one taking advantage of a situation, her actions excusable as simply out of her control and under the guise of innocence due to insanity. This is not only exhausting, but it is also troubling, as necessity for fatherly advice in this backdrop is an indication of severe decompensation, requiring a more one-sided line of questioning with subsequent stern advisement.

It's difficult to watch someone you have grown to care for give away the precious gift of self, especially in a state of instability complicated by a loss of appropriate judgement. I want to put her in the mental health hospital simply to keep her safe; however, criteria for dissolution of rights have not been truly met. A 5150 requires a person to be an imminent threat to self or others. At the very least, the criteria of grave disability must be met, and a person who drove themselves to an appointment and is appropriately groomed and showered would not make meeting such criteria realistic. I take very seriously the rights of others, and imposing an involuntary hold, even for just 72 hours, remains a state of suspension regarding a person's basic right to freedom. Against my often-blind inclination to protect, I make an agreement of sorts with Anna. We arrange weekly appointments until she is stabilized, and with such a contract, I do not push for inpatient admission.

As I see her every week following this decompensation, she walks into the room stating a number. In this, I am forced to devise an equation to measure the severity of her illness by the quantity of new sexual partners since our last assessment. I feel forced to watch another human being make sequential poor choices. Often these choices are not of her own accord. They are choices inspired and fueled by a mental illness.

As her mood begins to regulate, thankfully the number of sexual encounters also decreases. With this regulation comes clarity, and with it guilt for the recent encounters she engaged in. I am there now simply to comfort her through the guilt and shame followed by such numerous, and brazen, sexual acts. As coherence gives rise to insight upon the recent cracks in her moral parameters, I witness the subsequent depressive state. Her depressive symptoms become a proverbial cloud of darkness coaxing her to end her own life on a daily basis. For safety, we increase the frequency of her visits from once to twice per week. It turns out the unbridled mountain of sexuality is even less worrisome than the valley of hopelessness. Such hopelessness that is amplified in the shadow within recent states of grandiosity and elation.

Every meeting, every week, is a coaxing of safety and a mantra of positive thoughts of future change. For Anna, the suffering of bipolar depression encompasses thoughts of persistent plans and reasons to take her own life, and it takes all the energy I have to keep her alive during this time. It becomes a consistent search for the appropriate medication balance between her two polarities. Oftentimes, I am forced to use medications that most would never feel comfortable with in this patient population. I am at my wits' end, however, and willing to step out of my comfort zone to try unique therapies, all with the simple purpose of keeping my patient alive until she can stand up on her own and move forward. After months of concern and effort, along with weekly psychiatric follow-up appointments and countless medication alterations, we finally gather some semblance of the woman we knew before the storm, and with it, we slowly return to our normal banter.

Through Anna, I witnessed the most comprehensive symptom involvement for the disease we designate as bipolar disorder. In her alone, I witnessed the depth of presentations a patient with bipolar disorder can oscillate between. I witnessed her as an unassuming and genuinely sweet person, only to quickly transform to a highly irritable state, delivering verbal abuse to anyone in her line of sight. I witnessed her in a manic state laden with unbridled hypersexuality. She is a textbook example of bipolarity with states of mania equally reciprocated by periods of intense depression.

Together, Anna and I experienced firsthand the poles of her emotions. She would eventually prevail, winning the first battle of a never-ending war. Through her clearing, she would perform well for a time, but she would eventually learn to define happiness with elevated mood, as so many sufferers of mania express. She simply preferred to be in a state of energetic existence, and who could blame her when presented with the alternative. Thankfully, Anna did safely overcome her depression without any clear attempts on her life. She will, however, find herself in perpetual balance upon the tight rope of emotional regulation. Anna became the only patient that I could not anticipate. I would never be assured of a particular presentation during an upcoming outpatient appointment. It was a weekly game of roulette. I have a feeling that her saunter between divergent worlds of emotions may be her baseline level of function, and all I have to offer is support and an ever-watching eye.

CHAPTER 20

All the Pretty Dolls

BARBIE

"There's nothing worse than a man that can be everything to everybody else . . . except a father to their own child."
—Unknown

On day 4201, I meet Barbie. Barbie is a thin, 32-year-old Caucasian female with an obvious traumatic history. Her face is littered with sores indicative of chronic methamphetamine use only overshadowed by a trendy undercut hairstyle with both sides of the head shaved. This leaves the remaining locks on top in a state of isolation, ever confused on which way to fall. Her hairstyle seems to emulate the inner rejection of social norms. Maybe it's her way to give the middle finger to perceived norms and the society that failed her and betrayed her trust in every direction. Maybe it's her way to gain identity and uniqueness in a world seemingly overflowing with cattle in the ever-present herd mentality. It's also conceivable that her outward presentation is simply an unknowing tactic to be noticed, as the child inside her remains alone in a closet of loneliness with no one coming to her aid as she bangs on the proverbial door for help.

To the trained professional, history of trauma is often discernable on the face of its victims even when the individual attempts to hide behind a veil of euthymia. For others, these invisible scars lie hidden below the surface, and someone who does not know the individual to any great depth may never suspect such joy is actually an elusive presentation not representative of self. These blemishes of agony are often only noticeable with persistent conversation of topics comprising depth. Once the patient holds trust in you, then you may observe the lack of affective congruency throughout the reflection of trauma as well as the generalized absence of life in their eyes.

Of those young, carefree, and innocent girls exposed to trauma, many become consumed by guilt. Most, in one way or another, remain stifled in growth, blossoming to nothing but that of a fearful shell. They are often hypervigilant and remain guarded to admittance of harm for persistent fear of reprisal from their abuser. Some women may simply wish not to talk of such for fear of being perceived as weak or concerned that their story will not be deemed as valid or truthful. Individuals tortured by previous sexual and emotional trauma are not always blatantly suicidal, nor do they often present with active plans or intent to commit life-ending measures. Instead, they appear to almost search for death, taunting it, only by chance staying one step in front of Reaper's sickle. It's a test of death not by feats of glorious stunts or record-breaking attempts, but by the irresponsible choices and hazardous situations for which they place themselves. As is often the case, early traumatic history creates scarring of development, marring the sense of self and ever diminishing the ability to feel love, or deserved of such. This trauma provides a blow to the psyche, remaining continual and cancerous—an unforgiving course of metastasis affecting all aspects of the person's life.

Trauma can also obstruct the path to emotional maturity leading to an adult naïve to social concepts often taken for granted by others. This facilitates regression to a weakened immature state laden with child-like behaviors coupled with impulsive reactivity during times of stress or during exacerbations of emotional discourse. This seems to be the course of history that Barbie has been forced to struggle with.

My first assessment with Barbie began even before I realized it started. I witness her rush into the room only to jump and slide into the plastic chair across from me while providing a faint smile. She sits with both legs on the chair, resting her knees under her chin and wrapping her arms around her legs. She has a slight rocking motion back and forth, suddenly appearing shy and unwilling to make eye contact. Barbie appears frail and malnourished, sparking my will to feed her before any psychiatric interventions. Had my full-Italian grandmother been in the room, Barbie would have left five pounds heavier filled with pasta and bread and a pronounced urge to nap. Barbie is wearing the uniform of a meek, ragged, and beaten woman. She is fidgety and easily startled. Her county jail outfit, with the horizontal black-and-white-striped pattern, gives little addition of girth, as her form appears lost in the cloth. This vulnerable soul is now confined to jail, an environment of concrete and bars, all because of drug use and the poor choices that such a life initiated by trauma breeds.

"Tell me why you're here," I begin.

"Stealing." She hides her eyes with only a quick glance up to see what she expects to be another face of disappointment looking at her in judgement.

"Stealing? Like shoplifting, or did you rob someone?"

"Shoplifting," she says, replying with a drawn-out, careful tone with a volume only barely audible.

"Well, what did you steal? Anything good?" I attempt to lessen her anxiety, now apparent in the increased rapidity of her back-and-forth rocking.

"Just food," she replies. "I hadn't eaten in days."

"Okay." I contemplate my next words carefully and then just as quickly realize that's not my modus operandi. I just blurt things out with no filter. No need to alter my behavior now. "Stealing when you have nothing is understandable. I'm not saying you have the right to steal, ever, but if I was tempted with a meal to calm the pains of hunger, well,

I probably would have done the same thing." This garners a smile, while planting the seed of a fruitful, therapeutic relationship.

Knowing some details from her chart, I assume the homelessness reported on her last admission has changed little in her favor. "It must be hard to be homeless and hungry. I'm sorry you're having to deal with that type of situation. Maybe we can figure out a way to get you back on track." I truly have no idea what track she was once on and if it is even a track worth revisiting, but for now, I simply want to relay positivity and instill hope and drive for a better future.

She giggles and begins to sit up even straighter, the fear of judgement escaping her mind. "Everyone keeps laughing at me!" she says bluntly, like a child with ADHD (attention deficit hyperactivity disorder) who yells out possible answers during class.

"Who is laughing at you?" I ask.

"The other girls here. They always laugh 'cause I cry all the time and I pinch myself like this." She grabs the skin of her frail arm and pulls it farther than the pain should allow. "Sometimes I hear them laughing when no one is around. They follow me."

"How long have you been tormented by these voices?"

"Since I was a kid. I used to hear people talking and saying mean things to me but now it's mostly just laughing."

"So, you said you pinch yourself. Please tell me why you do this. Do you get a sense of relief?"

"Not really. It's a distraction from bad people."

"Okay, that makes sense." Patients love to be validated, and those four words do wonders to build trust. "So, the pain causes you to care little for the people and situations around you as all your mind can focus on is the discomfort. Do you feel like you deserve to be in pain?"

"Yes," she answers plainly with little regard to my wish for details.

"Why do you feel as though you deserve to be in pain?"

"I don't know." She shrugs her shoulders, her gaze once again fixed to the floor.

"I want to know why you're really here! Don't hold back! Look at me and tell me all the shit that has been done to you." I add the ingredient of inspiration she needs to elaborate on what I guessed was a rather chaotic past. I am not prepared for the story of suffering I hear at my own request and provocation.

"I killed my mother when I was seven."

I take a moment of silence. There is no book that teaches you what the hell to say when someone admits to murder. I attempt to soak in the statement and approach the situation with my left brain. I try to focus on the possibility that this may not be as it seems. After the appropriate time pondering, I take a deep breath and decide to play unfazed and simply continue with my questioning. "Tell me about this and why you feel you killed your mother."

"It was the day after Christmas, and I woke up, like, super tired from the previous day. I was still excited to play with my new Polly Pocket dollhouse. I can't believe I still remember that damn thing. As I was trying to rub the 'sleepies' from my eyes, I see my mother sitting on the edge of my bed crying. 'Mommy, did you stub your toe?' I asked her. I figured this was the case as I would often stub my toe climbing into bed 'cause my new bed frame was a solid wooden platform instead of the four-post frame I was used to. My mother shook her head and tried to wipe the tears away. I remember what happened next like it was yesterday. My mother looked and smiled at me like she had never done before. She told me she loved me, and I believed her. Maybe she did love me." Barbie pauses, obviously deciding if she is allowed to cry in this situation.

Not wanting to lose our progress, I continue to pry. "Tell me what happened next."

"She then told me to get her medicine for her nerves, which I easily recognized as I walked into her bathroom. I found the large yellow prescription bottle, the only one I had ever seen her use. I brought her the medicine like a good girl. She slowly took the bottle from my hands, opened it, and poured handful after handful, and just as quickly swallowed them till the bottle was empty on the bed next to her. I remember she laid back and said she was tired and needed to sleep. She was peacefully asleep, and I let her rest as I knew how grumpy she got when she was tired. I never knew how many methadone pills she took but it was a lot. All I know is that she never woke up. I didn't mean to kill her. She just laid down and died in front of me."

"You were seven, correct?"

"Yes."

"You were a small child then. Did you possess the strength to hold her nose closed while you fed those methadone pills into her mouth, as she struggled to overcome you?"

"No . . . it wasn't like that at all. She asked me to get her the pill bottle. When I gave it to her, she swallowed all of them."

"Let's get something straight real quick! Your mom ended her own life and you did nothing except be a great daughter and listen to what you were told to do. Take yourself out of the room, and out of the equation, and the story ends the same way. Do you understand what I am saying?"

"Yes, I do," she responds, her tone indicating that she does not want to accept my view yet understanding it's a key to the resolution of her guilt. Blame has most likely eaten at her, piece by piece, like a necrotizing bacterial infection. This infection has spread to all aspects of her life and she has accepted all that has been done to her after in a light of being deserved. Truth of what transpired that day after Christmas will be her antibiotic, ceasing any further spread such an infection of unwarranted responsibility can cause.

Throughout this entire initial assessment, she appears to be handling the recollection of her childhood trauma rather well. In fact, I am taken back by her command of language and the clarity of her speech. I'm impressed at the stoicism Barbie displays in the face of such a painful recollection. However, on closer inspection, I notice the right hand persistently pinching her left forearm, tugging and sharply pulling the skin as it lay crossed underneath the right arm. Her anxiety is bubbling to the surface as we move closer and closer to the most devastating of traumas she has yet to concede. Noticing her mood beginning to decompensate, I decide to terminate the interview. I analyze current and recent symptoms as well as previous psychiatric history, then prescribe the appropriate medications. At this point, it is time for the patient to rest.

I want to build the notion with her that sessions with me will not be long and tortuous but will consist of small insights into her past only so we can progress to the present symptoms and their management. I revert to my rule of, if we need to explore a traumatic past, we do it once, and we do it together. After that, we accept it as in the past and that it is something that cannot be altered or fixed. It doesn't even have to be something we understand. We correct any cognitive distortions of misunderstanding and continue to press forward. I do not believe that living in the past can heal what currently ails an individual. Sometimes, we just need to accept it as history and let it live or die in that same history. Taking agony, regret, and trauma with us throughout life only leads to more sorrow and leaves a part of us in the past unable to benefit and appreciate the future ahead.

Barbie returns to my office two days later, day 4,203, and I see in her a woman with a somewhat improved affect from our initial introduction.

After a few pleasantries and generalized questions, we continue where we initially left off. "Tell me what happened after your mother died."

"Well, I had no father, at least none that I ever met, so I was sent off to live with my mom's brother, my uncle Sam. Sam was married to Jeanie, who was a nice and loving lady, but she traveled for work quite frequently. Even when she was home, she was either oblivious to what was going on, or just didn't want to know. My therapist thinks she found comfort in denial. I don't know about all that, but because she was away so often, my uncle and I were forced to spend a lot of alone time together. It's strange 'cause he used to tell me I was the daughter he never had, yet looking back I wonder if he also blamed me for his sister's death. Maybe he used the blame as an excuse for the torture he put me through over the next seven years until I could muster up enough energy as a fourteen-year-old to run away for life on the streets."

I cautiously continue forward, trying to understand the pain she endured. "Tell me more, please, but know we can stop at any time you begin to feel uncomfortable."

"I was seven when he started locking me in the hallway closet. He would tell me over and over that 'all the pretty dolls stay in the closet.'" She pauses, looking to the corner of the room, possibly determining if she wants to stop the interview. However, she appears to build strength with every word uttered to a listening ear.

"I always knew I was in for it when I would hear people come to the door. After a few minutes of whispering, my uncle would open the closet and grab my arm. He would stick a needle in me, which I later learned was heroin. I guess they thought if I was doped up, I wouldn't remember. Then he would let random men go to the closet, carry me into my bedroom, and have their way with me. These pieces of shit would often beat me in the process of raping me. Of course, my uncle would say, 'They are just getting their money's worth. When you get older, you're going to give it away for free anyway. Stop whining, and if you don't fight back, you won't get hurt.' I later learned he was actually trading me to fuel his heroin habit."

She begins to tremble as her lips tighten over clenched teeth and matching fists. Her tears display an emotional dysregulation, an odd mixture of anger and sadness reserved only for humans.

If we were to look at her from a neurological perspective at this immediate point, we would see overactivity in the amygdala, the part of the brain that deals with emotion. At the same time, blood flow is increasing to the frontal lobe, specifically the part of the brain that's over the left eye. This area controls reasoning and is likely what's keeping her from all-out-rage in my office. These areas generally balance each other out, quickly diffusing our immediate response to attack in the lacking presence of a charging bear. The brain is typically able to restructure the acute fight-or-flight response, yet this has little to do with the part of the brain responsible for harboring memories that can continue to trigger responses of fury.

This story of childhood innocence lost, and of purity being traded for drugs, is obviously particularly hard to hear. I keep telling myself this is about her and that I must stay strong for her. I try my best to stay in the moment and not let my emotions overwhelm my professional manner.

Just as I am about to terminate the interview, Barbie makes the oddest of comments. She looks at me and states, "I feel bad for Minnie. She got the worst of it."

"Who is Minnie?" I ask, thinking I must have overlooked a sibling throughout the story.

"Minnie is what they used to call me when I was younger. Minnie wants revenge! I try to tell her no, but she is stronger and I'm not always able to control her. Sometimes she wins and takes over."

It's altogether possible that "Minnie" was the name she was called when she was younger or it may simply be a name derived by Barbie as a coping mechanism, a name that allows her a conduit to the anger and memories of pain. Minnie may be a way for her to deflect responsibility or she may be the safety of dissociation allowing her to feel sorry for someone else rather than accepting that such acts were done to her.

Through further investigation, I realize Minnie is a constant presence, a persistent voice, not in her head but in its own space seemingly coming from a person next to her. This person is without form, with no measurable mass, but is just as real as the mind will allow. Minnie has shared memories yet different forms of coping mechanism. Minnie appears to be less innocent and much more violent than her alter ego based in reality. Minnie is the form looking to gain power, to protect herself and inflict pain on those who threatened her. Barbie remains in an immature and naïve state, while Minnie has learned protection and perseverance through anger and violence. The regression in Barbie's maturity to her pre-pubescent self is seamless, and oddly in the third person. The secondary identity seems to be less distinct and more of a scapegoat for thoughts of violent intent, influenced by the patient's emotional state.

After some very strange and murderously detailed responses, Minnie quickly presents to be the self that could enact revenge in an attempt to regain the innocence she lost—innocence she felt could be earned through the power of violence. I cautiously surmise that Barbie may be suffering from a state of dissociative identity disorder (DID). A complex diagnosis of such, however, would require extensive, future evaluations, and the time for such is not something I am provided in this environment of "treat and release."

Multiple personality disorder (MPD) has been recently renamed DID in the latest version of the psychiatric based *Diagnostic and Statistical Manual of Mental Disorders* (DSM). The disorder of DID is a realization of the complexity and rarity provided by such a diagnosis. This controversial diagnosis was first brought to the mainstream by the best-selling book *Sybil*. The book portrayed the story of a young woman plagued with multiple personalities and was sold as a detailed account as provided to her psychiatrist. After the book was published in 1973, it blossomed with a mainstream movie portrayal of the book under the same name. The prevalence of this once rare disorder began to climb. Was this due to the increased awareness of the disorder or due to the provocative complexity such a disorder conveys?

It was later discovered that the symptoms specific to Sybil's case may have been a distortion of the truth and possibly nothing more than fiction. This is not to say that DID doesn't exist, as some psychiatrists believe, but may be extensively rare in our current understanding. What we can know is that the case of Sybil may have been more indicative of a study of the impressionable mind under the influence of drugs and hypnosis. The patient we call Sybil was regularly injected with sodium pentothal, which was then being used to help people remember repressed traumatic events. Under the influence of drugs and hypnosis, the very suggestible Sybil provided her many personalities, all under the coercion of her physician motivated to develop such personalities to create a fictional tale of a very real condition. This physician was possibly attempting to gain notice and affirmation above the wellness of his patient. It is situations such as this, and many more vile tales, that have given the field of psychiatry its tortured past and corrupt reputation. As a result, it is a specialty trying to redefine itself with the practice of only using methods related to evidenced-based studies.

Securing a diagnosis of DID is difficult even for the most experienced of clinicians and not something I was prepared to do at this time in my training. All that mattered was that to Barbie, Minnie was real, and maybe this wasn't all bad. Maybe this alter ego was a source of strength for her, and if she was able to focus such strength without the violence accompanying Minnie, maybe she could grow to stand on her own, looking upon the future with hope realizing she is not defined by the trauma she has suffered. I hope that she viewed her trauma as being the worst life has to offer, and that she still survived and overcame. I hope she would one day flourish into the woman she was destined to be.

I was, however, left in wonderment of the human mind and its attempts to guard consciousness from severe traumas. All I could do was attempt to treat the symptoms presenting in Barbie's current condition and hope to guide her towards inspiration of self-love. I wanted to replace that fragile shell with strength and resolve. I wanted her to see the woman of great potential that I saw seated before me. A woman greater than the sum of her traumas.

I often wondered about the woman she may have become had she been provided with a loving home. I knew no amount of therapy or psychopharmacology could ever revive her innocence or dissolve the torture she was forced to endure. Barbie was the first patient that ever forced me to realize my limitations. That day, in my car, I gave myself to a greater power and prayed. I prayed for her future and swift release from the torment inside. I prayed for knowledge and guidance to help her. I prayed that the men that brutally abused her were found by their transgressions and were forced to pay for what evils they had committed. I prayed for Barbie to simply find sanctity and happiness in whatever life could be pieced together.

CHAPTER 21

Look, Mom!

MATTHEW

"Paranoid? Probably. But just because you're paranoid doesn't mean there isn't an invisible demon about to eat your face."
—Jim Butcher

Imagine sitting in the movie theatre with your two best friends. The smell of popcorn is filling all your senses. The lights dim, inviting the movie to finally commence. Through the previews, you gasp and smile, making mental notes of the movies your future self may enjoy. The feature begins and all seems enjoyable at first. You sink into your chair, ready to be taken out of your reality, when you slowly begin to witness patterns eerily similar to your own life. You start to make connections that are too random to be left to coincidence. Each character represents someone in your life, and with each moment, you become more and more convinced that something is amiss as for this to be merely chance would be implausible.

Paranoia starts to settle in, and with it, your heart begins to race. Those buttery, popcorn-stained hands become ever clammier as you start to perspire. Looking cautiously to the left and right, you check to see if anyone recognizes that this movie is about your life. You begin to scan the auditorium knowing that some, if not all, of these individuals must be in on it. Not sure if this is a set-up or a warning, you become ever-more alert. The dark theatre begins to close in and feels more like a coffin. Hypervigilance envelopes your thought process. Your heart rate rises and begins to race, providing the feeling as though it is going to jump out of your chest. The epinephrine-induced fight-or-flight response is now in full evolutionary representation.

You become certain that your suspicions are intact and that this must be a plot to flush you out. Aware of the impending danger, you slowly stand up, making no mention to your "friends," as you assume, they must be part of the plot as well, being that this was their idea. You move down the aisle, stepping slowly as to not draw attention, yet fast enough to limit the exposure. With your left hand raised to cover your face, you continue down the stairs to the ground level. Reaching the bottom, you quickly turn right and down the hall towards the exit. You finally reach the concession stand of the theatre and take a deep breath. Knowing the danger has only temporarily ceased, you plan your escape.

Cautiously walking, with head down, you reach the outermost doors of the theatre. Here you begin to run for safety, and with no particular sense of direction, you quickly become overwhelmed by the darkness. With the fear that the next passing car will be the hitman sent to fulfill an execution, you dart into the orange groves adjacent to the expressway. Here, you find comfort in the absence of light.

After cautiously removing the phone from your pocket, you call the only person you're certain you can trust. When you hear the comfort of your mother's voice, your sequestered emotions overwhelm you. In a frantic state, you purge all your current ideals of paranoia, maintaining that unknown people are out to get you. She can hardly make sense of the accusations you present and urges you to call the police. You comply, and while on the phone with the 911 dispatcher, you lie in hiding. With your chest to the dirt, you pray the cavalry reaches you before those who wish you harm discover your location.

You remain prone, cautiously awaiting confirmation of the calvary. After a good period of time without relief, you begin to venture further into the rows of citrus to seek your own path to safety. Reaching a farmhouse, you knock firmly on the glass front door, hoping to find some consolation of protection inside. With every passing moment paranoia increases, and in unfamiliar territory, reality begins to blur. With the persistent slippage of reason, you presume there must be persons inside the farmhouse that are in danger. What other reason would they have for not answering your pleas? In an attempt to free the inhabitants from this potential unspoken threat, you quickly devised a plan to break them out of the house. Transitioning from prey to savior, you decide to break in and carry the inhabitants to safety. You slam both arms into the window adjacent to the front door and your arms find their way easily through the glass. You retract them to reach the lock and, in such motion, shred the flesh from your arms as they peel against the jaded glass shards still clinging to the window frame. You fall to the floor of the porch in agony and rest in a pool of your own blood as the owners of the home cower in fear for their own lives. Savior and prey now all similarly bracing for police response.

In the emergency department, the patient required STAT trauma and vascular surgery to repair lacerations to the left ulnar artery, right radial artery, and right ulnar artery. The surgery required arterial bypass using the saphenous vein as a graft. He also required a rather large skin graft from his right thigh to cover the exposed damage and dramatic loss of skin of the right wrist and forearm.

It's day 4,198, and upon walking into the room, I see a group of nursing students working on fresh bandages on a patient's left hand, using his severe injury as a learning opportunity on how to care for patients after skin graft, vascular surgery, and general mayhem. His mother is present at the end of his bed comfortably seated in a hospital chair. She stands upright with her hand outstretched for a greeting as I walk into the room. She obviously became a mother at a relatively early age as she doesn't look a day older than me. Her skin-tight red dress leaves little to the imagination, hugging every curve of her body. Decorated with a white shoal and matching high heels, she introduces herself. Obviously, she is a woman who likes the attention and is used to getting whatever and whomever she sets her sights on.

After our introduction, she gestures to the patient in the medical bed. "This is my son, Matthew. We appreciate you coming by. He could really use your help."

Turning to the man of the hour, I see a young, slender chap of 20 years lying in bed. Matthew, like his mother, also appears younger than his stated age. If I was to see him on the street, I would assume he was maybe 16, and certainly not close to legal drinking age.

He lies motionless in bed with his head slightly propped up. Both arms are in bandages, with braces over each forearm and wrist to limit any movement. Although in this precarious state of self-inflicted trauma, he lies content, adorning a huge smile most likely due to the attention of the female nursing students.

I was forewarned that he was severely upset regarding his newly labeled condition of schizophrenia. Being a gifted student, he has the insight to realize what such a diagnosis entails and the limitations that are often inescapable. He knows this would be the end of his formulated goals and aspirations. However, I believe the diagnosis was potentially given prior to historical knowledge of the course of his illness, so I keep an open mind for alternative theories.

After pleasantries, I begin my assessment. I open with his mother, gathering collateral about his performance in school and his social life. She details a highly motivated and gifted student who is adored by many friends. The prom king, the president of student government; a boy ever active in the community. She discusses his artistic talents and reiterates his drive and ability for sustained energy.

I turn to Matthew, believing his mother's short description may be indicative of another condition altogether. "So, I heard you're not happy about finding out you have schizophrenia."

His smile is released from duty and he becomes saddened. "No, not at all."

"Well, I have some good news for you. I don't think you have schizophrenia."

"Really?" He raises his head above the pillows, now fixated on the present conversation.

"Let me ask you some questions so we can figure out what's going on. I'm going to guess you have difficulty sleeping. Also, you experience periods of time when you only sleep two or three hours per night but still awaken feeling fully rested."

"I do."

"Do these episodes last for about a week?"

"Yeah, or longer." I can hear initiations of excitement growing in his voice.

"During the same time as you're having these severe sleep disturbances, do you get really motivated to start multiple projects, often starting multiple unique undertakings without ever finishing them?"

"That's exactly what happens."

"I'm also going to guess that during these times of multiple project development, you feel amazing! You feel like the smartest man on the planet. You become intensely focused, yet you feel like your mind is racing. Also, during these times, you are told by people you interact with that you are talking too much or too fast."

"Oh my God, that is me!"

"That describes him perfectly," his mother adds, now standing next to me.

"That's exactly me!" he responds again, reiterating his case and now with the previous smile reaffixed on his face.

"Well, those are all symptoms of something called bipolar disorder. It's a disorder that we can treat, and if you stay adherent to medications, you can enjoy a long and fruitful life."

"So, I'm not schizophrenic?"

"No, you are certainly not."

"Yes!" he yells out. He raises both arms high above his head in victory and screams, "Look, Mom. I'm bipolar!" His reaction is similar in elation as if he had just hit the lottery. He is so excited nothing could suffice other than a scream while raising both hands to the sky.

I can't help but smile and laugh. "Yes, you are."

We continue to chat about bipolar disorder, its treatments, and expectations. He is yet again a patient defined by the name of his diagnosis. These diagnoses to patients are not just letters strung together in sequence but those of having the purpose to gauge severity of impending doom. That is why, with each patient, I discuss their diagnosis in detail, and I always give them the opportunity to label themselves with whatever diagnosis they see fit, as long as the treatment modalities are that of similar substances associated with my perception of their diagnosis.

I give Matthew a list of very creative and famous people with reported bipolar disorder. This only further excites his state of self, feeling proud to be in the company of such great men and women. He and his mother, as well as I, all agree to a treatment strategy of temporary antipsychotics with long-term maintenance found through mood stabilizers such as Depakote or Lithium.

Patients often need to know their diagnosis. They feel compelled to learn the name of their demons. This diagnosis may be beneficial to the patient if it cements the necessity for medication adherence. Sometimes, however, the diagnosis that follows them becomes a weight too intense to bear, one that has the potential to create isolation for fear of stigma as well as devouring the confidence to follow their goals and aspirations. A diagnosis can be defeating, and in those patients, we should tread carefully and worry more about presenting symptoms and clinical presentations than determining what box to fit the patient into.

Although our time together was short, I will never forget Matthew or his reaction to his newfound diagnosis. He serves as a perfect example of the dangers placing the permanence of a diagnosis can create before sufficient and extensive rule outs. I often imagine Matthew happy and successful. I believe he will learn to focus his mania and with it have the gift of increased energy, focus, and drive.

I can envision his success guided by his diagnosis rather than restricted by such. I can picture him walking across the stage of his college graduation with a bright smile and his arms raised high in success, yelling down to his family, "Look, Mom. I did it!"

CHAPTER 22

Conclusion

FIGHTING THE STIGMA

Increased awareness about mental health is emerging in society, yet a stigma shadowing mental health disorders, the labels affixed, and patients suffering from such still resides. Stigma refers to the condition in which someone judges another depending on a singular and particular personality trait. It's a way to discount all that makes us unique, and it reduces us down to a worth, or lack thereof, based solely on our imperfections.

Society in general is plagued with preconceived notions concerning what is believed to be true regarding mental illness. A great percentage of this stigma originates from sources of dramatization, such as seen in movies and television shows. Very little true and accurate information regarding mental illness, and psychiatry, is available to the curious navigator, and much less the ill-informed societal participant who receives most of the breaking news at the checkout stand in their local grocery store.

With the inception of the internet and platforms of social networking, information, either true, false, or simply embellished, spreads easily and profusely. Unfortunately, shocking news, like news about the crazed individual with mental health issues, are the news stories that most can equate to an experience of psychiatric disorders. If all we hear or experience in this information age are stories of mental health illness being the inciting factor in mass shootings and murderous inclinations, then it may be hard to blame individuals exposed for propagating such a stigma. "If it bleeds, it leads," as the famous saying goes regarding which stories gain front page precedence.

Those with mental illness have found no open arms to recovery but instead are labeled as dangerous, impulsive, and unpredictable. Much of how an individual perceives mental illness is based upon their own personal experience with such conditions. Someone who has seen their loved one suffer with a mental health disorder is much more likely to recognize the illness as not so different than any other illness of the body. Most people with mental health disorders are not dangerous. They are not sociopathic individuals roaming the streets at night searching for unsuspecting victims. They are your neighbors, your child's teacher, your brother, sister, or they may even be you. The only reason they remain hidden is because we have given them no light to step in to.

In our society today, people are fixated on labels and appearances. People with mental health issues, regardless of the severity, will deliberately avoid being "marked" as having a psychiatric disorder. These individuals prefer to suffer in silence simply to avoid the backlash that comes from such a label being placed within their defined identity.

I once had an overtly anxious woman come to my office just ripe and ready for an argument. She had suffered the stigma of mental illness, and her last psychiatrist had given her a diagnosis she didn't agree with and, according to her, was unwilling to waver on his designation in her electronic medical record. I listened patiently as she spoke of her transgressions of not being heard by medical providers. When she was done expressing her frustration, she displayed a puzzled look, as I had not given the reaction, or defensive posture, she had assumed I would provide.

Instead, I looked at her and said, "I see here in the chart it states that you have schizoaffective disorder depressive type." I turn the screen to show her what she already knew to be true. She began in on her rant again when I interrupted her. "What do you think your diagnosis is?"

"Well, I think it's major depressive disorder with psychotic features," she quickly and confidently responded.

I fell quiet again, turning the computer screen back to my view. She waited quietly as I hit a few keys of the keyboard and used my mouse to make a few clicks. I turned the computer screen back to her and showed her that I erased the previous diagnosis and imputed MDD with psychotic features. "Now your diagnosis is MDD with psychotic features."

Her draw dropped, her eyes swelled, and she immediately said, "How did you do that?"

"I am here not to label you, nor to fit you into one of eight boxes on my screen. I don't care what your diagnosis is. You are in charge of your own care, and your label, or lack thereof, will not change how I treat you."

All the intense frustration she had carried on her back for years was gone. She had finally been listened to. Of course, my treatment would have been the same regardless of which of the two diagnoses was chosen, but to her, the label mattered. To her, what others read about her diagnosis or thought about her on a personal level was now up to her and of her choosing. We had two years together with an outstanding therapeutic relationship that lasted until my residency was over. This was not because I was so different than the rest and not because I was more clever or intelligent. Our relationship was based on getting her involved in her own care. Our relationship was not about affixing a label of disease but caring for the person, a real human person who simply happened to be suffering from a psychiatric disorder.

It is no secret that mental illness is surrounded by stigma. There are numerous negative terms used to describe people with mental illness, and many of these terms are used in everyday conversation. We have become so complacent with such labels that most have no idea that they are furthering the stigma by using them. Instead of perpetuating conviction, deliberately or otherwise, we must stand together to accept those with mental illness, not in a light of judgement but instead as another human being suffering from an illness outside their control. Only once the stigma of mental illness is lifted will we as a society progress to an empathetic understanding of the torment others face.

"If you judge people, you have no time to love them."
Mother Teresa

Made in the USA
Monee, IL
04 November 2026

67383306R00207